the
healthy skin
kitchen

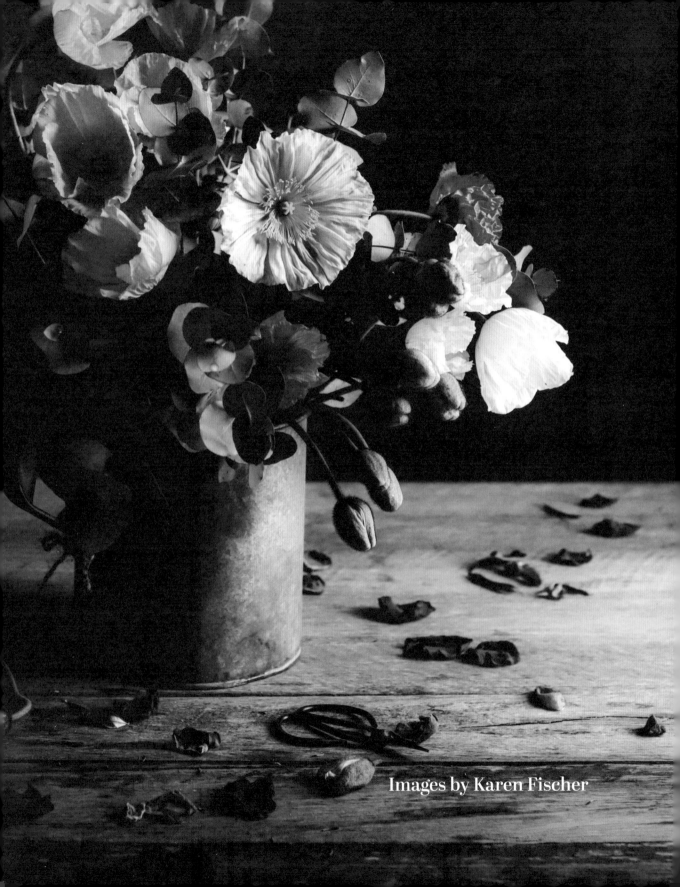

Images by Karen Fischer

the
healthy skin
kitchen

FOR ECZEMA, DERMATITIS, PSORIASIS, ACNE, ALLERGIES, HIVES,
ROSACEA, RED SKIN SYNDROME, CELLULITE, LEAKY GUT, MCAS,
SALICYLATE SENSITIVITY, HISTAMINE INTOLERANCE & MORE

KAREN FISCHER   BHSc, Dip. Nut.

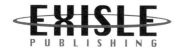

EXISLE
PUBLISHING

About the author

Karen Fischer is an Australian nutritionist who holds a Bachelor of Health Science Degree. With a love of nutritional biochemistry and a passion for nutrition, over the past twenty years Karen has created various food programs to help thousands of people with real skin issues.

Karen has penned six health books including the best-sellers *The Eczema Detox*, *The Eczema Diet* and the award-winning book *The Healthy Skin Diet* (Australian Food Media Awards, 2008). In the 1990s Karen was a popular children's television presenter and in 2008 the media went crazy for her tips on marketing healthy food to children. She has appeared on Sky News, Seven's *Sunrise* and *Today Tonight*, Nine Network's *A Current Affair*, *What's Up Doc?* and *The Morning Show* and in 2014 Karen's 'breakthrough diet for eczema' story appeared on primetime Seven News. Karen has written various articles for *The Sun Herald*, *Body+Soul* and *Madison* magazine and she had a health column in *Cosmopolitan* magazine.

Karen now spends her time running a company called Skin Friend, developing products to help people love their skin and enjoy life. When she is not wearing hats, you'll find her cooking in the kitchen or lying on a yoga mat. She has two beautiful children and lives a quiet life by the beach.

Karen's websites and social media include:
www.skinfriend.com
www.eczemalife.com
www.healthyskinkitchen.com
@skinfriend.co

Praise

Dear Karen,

Where do I start? I have always suffered from eczema. I remember as a child being jealous of other kids in assembly who had smooth skin on the backs of their knees while mine were all scabby and sore. Throughout my life I have had good and bad times, including nearly being put in hospital in my early twenties as I had hypothermia due to the rawness of my skin and I looked like a burns victim. I have tried so many diets and creams and used steroids for years but never really managed to get on top of it.

Leading up to Christmas 2017 my skin was bad, so as a New Year's resolution I started on what I thought would be a healthy diet: no dairy, alcohol or chocolate but lots of fresh fruit and vegetables, lean meats etc. But I went from bad to worse, I was covered from head to toe with eczema and itched like crazy. The doctor put me on stronger steroid creams, prednisone and antihistamines day and night but I saw little improvement. I was signed off work for a month to see if it was stress-related but only saw a small improvement. The doctor recommended me to a skin specialist and while waiting I found your book, supplements and website.

I was very sceptical, given I had tried so many diets before, but I had to do something. I was so unwell I had nothing to lose. The results were amazing — within ten days I was able to stop taking the antihistamines, it felt like coming out of a fog, the itching was reducing. The skin specialist wanted me to try drugs to suppress my immune system usually used for a certain type of cancer treatment and this meant a two-year course with the possibility of some side effects. As I was beginning to see some improvements to my skin by following your diet, we agreed to delay taking the drugs.

I followed your diet for five months and by the following Christmas my skin was eczema-free and I had lost that bit of extra weight I could never shift, even though I was eating lots of food and never hungry while on your diet. Over a year later I am still eczema-free. Thank you again, you have changed my life, my skin is the best it has ever been and so smooth. The healing power of your diet is amazing.

KATE SMITH, NEW ZEALAND

The Healthy Skin Kitchen is a visual feast and a heartfelt guide to skin wellness. I greatly value and prioritize health and wellbeing in my life and this book will serve as a wonderful guide to anyone who wants to maintain a healthy diet whilst allowing their skin to reap the benefits. As a former patient and close friend for 27 years, I trust Karen's advice and her recipes are delicious!

—MEGAN GALE, MODEL, MOTHER, ACTRESS AND BUSINESSWOMAN

This sublime book is much more than a recipe book. It's a work of art. Karen Fischer's gentle wisdom interweaved with cutting edge research on skin health and sublime photographs compel you to convert to the healthy eating way.

—JACINTA TYNAN, JOURNALIST AND AUTHOR

Karen knows first-hand the pain, discomfort and debilitation chronic skin issues can have on your life. As an award-winning author, nutritionist and health expert, Karen provides a warm and insightful look into her and her daughter's journey with skin issues, and provides the healthy and delicious recipes she created to heal them. The best part is all of the recipes are customizable, so if you have an issue with a particular ingredient, Karen provides delicious alternatives, which is helpful as you will literally want to eat all of the meals right off the page.

—ALICE HAMPTON, ACP MANAGEMENT AND FORMER VICE PRESIDENT OF GLOBAL
COMMUNICATIONS FOR SHISEIDO AND BAREMINERALS

Praise for Karen's other books

The Healthy Skin Diet
Thank you so much for a concise and well researched book. If I said it's changed my life I would sound clichéd, but that sums it up. I'm 31 and have suffered from acne since I was fifteen. It's been six days and I can honestly say I've seen better results than in a decade of trying. Much love and appreciation.

—CAMILLA

The Eczema Diet
I am 51 years of age and have suffered from eczema since I was around three years old. So now I have followed the guidelines of Karen's book. In the last six months my progress has much improved. My 'flare ups' are not as aggressive and do not last as long. The swelling

has gone down and is not as red, no more weepy skin on my neck and eyelids. I can get water on my face! I don't have crying temper tantrums when my hands, face and neck are so itchy I'm scratching them raw. I'm getting more than two hours sleep a night, sometimes even 6! *Yaaah.* My sheets and pillow slips are not constantly in the wash. These are just a few of the improvements. I've still got a wee way to go but it's nice to see a little light at the end of such a very long, depressing and dark tunnel. Thank you Karen.

—AMANDA THOMPSON, NEW ZEALAND

My son, who is now one, has had eczema since he was three months old. I started eliminating foods in the hope that would be the answer. I found Karen's book *The Eczema Diet* and started implementing parts of her diet — adjusting it to my son's multitude of food allergies — and his eczema started to clear. When he turned one, I was able to start giving him AM and PM supplements. Can I just say, *game changer!* Karen, thank you for being a part of my son's journey to health!

—LINDSEY ANDERSON, UNITED STATES

I am so thankful for your book *The Eczema Diet* that I wanted to write and tell you how much it has helped us. I used to worry that my daughter would not be able to get married and have children because her hands were so, so sore. She could barely look after herself — she wouldn't have been able to look after a home or a baby. But during the year we were on the Eczema Diet, she met the man she would marry. By their wedding day she was completely cured with beautiful skin, and now they are joyfully expecting their first child. *Beat that for a happy ending!*

—TANI NEWTON, NEW ZEALAND

The Eczema Detox
This book has really helped heal my eczema and psoriasis. I am doing the FID Program and am testing foods currently. It's been life changing!

—CATHERINE JOHNSON, UNITED STATES (AMAZON.COM REVIEW)

After two years of struggling with painful rosacea and spending $$$$, this diet was a welcome relief. It's hard to commit to, but once I did, I saw results right away. Read all the material, follow the recipes, and you won't regret it.

—ALEXA, CANADA (AMAZON.COM REVIEW)

First published 2021

Exisle Publishing Pty Ltd
PO Box 864, Chatswood, NSW 2057, Australia
226 High Street, Dunedin, 9016, New Zealand
www.exislepublishing.com

A CiP record for this book is available from the National Library
of Australia.

ISBN 978 1 925820 65 2

Designed by Mark Thacker
Typeset in Miller Text Roman 10 on 15pt
Printed in China

This book uses paper sourced under ISO 14001 guidelines from
well-managed forests and other controlled sources.

10 9 8 7 6 5 4 3 2 1

Disclaimer
This book is a general guide only and should never be a substitute
for the skill, knowledge and experience of a qualified medical
professional dealing with the facts, circumstances and symptoms
of a particular case. The nutritional, medical and health information presented in this book is based on the research, training and
professional experience of the author, and is true and complete
to the best of their knowledge. However, this book is intended
only as an informative guide; it is not intended to replace or
countermand the advice given by the reader's personal physician.
Because each person and situation is unique, the author and the
publisher urge the reader to check with a qualified healthcare
professional before using any procedure where there is a ques-
tion as to its appropriateness. The author, publisher and their
distributors are not responsible for any adverse effects or conse-
quences resulting from the use of the information in this book. It
is the responsibility of the reader to consult a physician or other
qualified healthcare professional regarding their personal care.
This book contains references to products that may not be available everywhere. The intent of the information provided is to be
helpful; however, there is no guarantee of results associated with
the information provided.

Contents

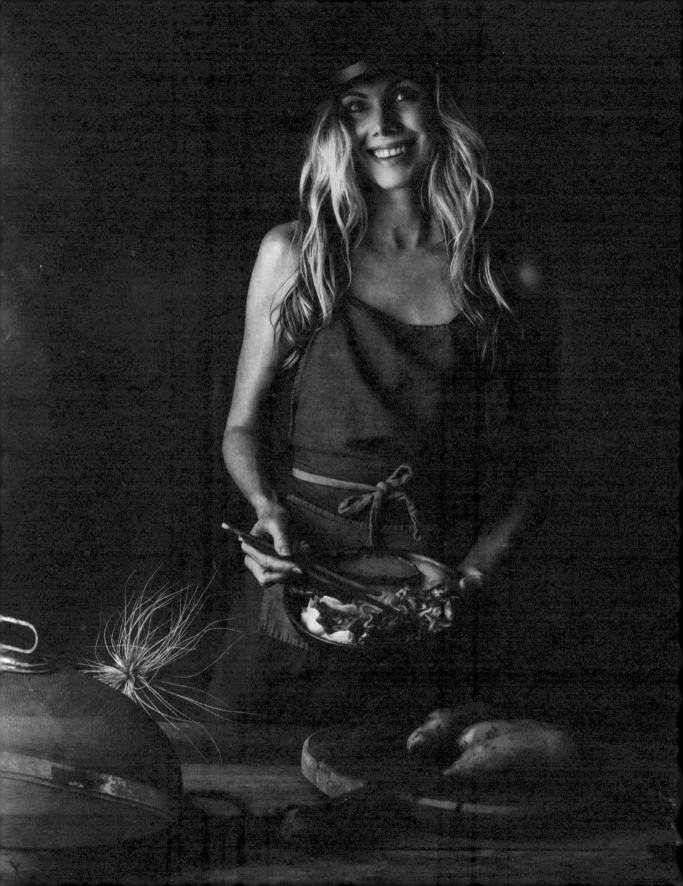

Introduction

They say when life gives you lemons, make a margarita (or something like that). For me, life gave me skin issues. And I have suffered some of the worst, including head-to-toe eczema, hives, psoriasis, rosacea, dermatitis, breakouts and severe multiple chemical intolerances that left me unable to eat much at all. As an adult, I have been in despair and so damn itchy that I could not sleep for days. So if you are going through anything difficult right now, I get it. It's embarrassing and painful and don't get me started on the social isolation.

Skin issues seem to run in my family too. My daughter Ayva was born with eczema and she became the inspiration for my journey into skin wellness more than twenty years ago. Ayva is also the reason I wrote *The Eczema Diet*. But that was a long time ago ... Today she is twenty and has beautiful skin and she lives a normal life so I'm really thankful for that.

Before I was a nutritionist I was always on the hunt for topical products that could help my skin. I found store-bought products either stung my skin, gave me pimples or they weren't hydrating enough — my skin was painfully dry, especially in winter, and seriously nothing helped. So out of necessity I learnt how to make my own skin creams. Word grew and soon my cousins, aunties and uncles who suffered from crazy dry, flaky skin (like me) were testing my homemade concoctions. And the feedback was promising ... After trying one of my rescue balms for a week my Auntie Merle, who is 83, said, 'I'm Benjamin Button: I'm ageing backwards'. So we put her in a home (just kidding, but I did use her quote when the product went online).

It really feels like my whole life has led me towards the field of skin health and while I don't really like mentioning my age, I've got to say that being 47 has been surprisingly good. After having flaky skin for most of my life and a serious case of eczema, I now marvel at how baby soft my skin looks and feels: I'm truly amazed at my skin's ability to heal and renew and change. And when I wake up in the morning with clear skin (after a good night's sleep!) I say thank you and remind myself how wonderful life is. Today I feel incredibly grateful to be able to share my tips, recipes and twenty years of expertise with you. Welcome to my cooking adventure ...

About the book

As a curious nutritionist, I have tried and tested many popular diets and skin care products (sometimes to the detriment of my skin). I have been a dedicated vegan, a pescatarian and I dabbled in autoimmune paleo after my immune system went psycho (hello stress response!). And while health experts might try to box you into one cure-all diet (that does not exist), I have learnt that one size does *not* fit all so my recipes are skewed towards skin health, utilizing relevant aspects of my favourite tried-and-tested diets.

- » If you value veganism or need to eat autoimmune paleo in order to feel well, you can find Healthy Skin Kitchen (HSK) recipes and menus that are in line with your values and/or health needs.
- » All of the recipes are dairy-free and many are gluten-free for those who need to avoid gluten.
- » There are instructions on how to adapt the recipes for those with food intolerances.
- » And my recipes are low–moderate in salicylates and histamines, because I have seen the miracles a low chemical diet can produce when it comes to healing chronic skin inflammation and leaky gut.

What I am about to share with you is a new way of eating that has firmed and toned and repaired my skin like no other diet has ever done before. It's based on the programs I have used to help my patients and family over the past twenty years, plus exciting new research and additional recipes. And the best bit is it's tailored to you.

Foods that bite: What is a low chemical diet?

I feel the need to keep speaking out about chemical intolerance as the scientific research is continually ignored by health practitioners and bloggers alike, so people continue to suffer needlessly with skin (and gut) symptoms that could be alleviated with a low-chemical diet.

What is a low chemical diet and why should you try it?

You may have heard of *chemical sensitivity* or *chemical intolerance*. If you are sensitive to chemicals you might adversely react to perfumes, household cleaning products and the chlorine in your pool. You might also be sensitive to food colourings, artificial flavourings and preservatives. Many health-conscious people avoid artificial additives and chemical cleaning products and believe they are living a low chemical lifestyle. But with the rise in popularity of fermented foods, cacao, turmeric and red wine, people are ingesting incredible amounts of natural chemicals called histamines and salicylates, which can lead to a different type of toxicity. People can suffer for years with chemical toxicity symptoms and never know it's certain foods that are making them sick. Symptoms such as pain, inflammation, fatigue, eczema, hives and other skin rashes, sinusitis, rosacea, psoriasis, hay fever, migraines, ADHD, arthritis, IBS, bloating and other signs of leaky gut, can be worsened or triggered by excess ingestion of histamines, salicylates and other chemicals, both natural and artificial. The body in an autoimmune response can also make excess histamine, so this book addresses this too.

How do you know if *food chemical intolerance* is triggering your symptoms? You'll never know unless you try a low chemical diet

If you would like a free 'food chemical chart' where you can look up any ingredient and see the content of histamines, amines and salicylates, join my newsletter at skinfriend.com and the PDF will be automatically emailed to you (the newsletter sign-up box is at the bottom of the website).

to see how your body responds. So, if you find that this book does not include a favourite trendy ingredient (such as cacao, turmeric or fermented foods), it's because it's either too rich in histamines, salicylates and/or glutamates such as MSG. These natural chemicals are not necessarily bad for you but their *overconsumption* can lead to health problems when your body's detoxification systems become overwhelmed. Your liver can only cope with so much work before it becomes depleted in nutrients — the result is food intolerances, allergies and a range of symptoms that gradually worsen. Following a nourishing, low chemical diet gives your liver and gastrointestinal tract a much-needed break from chemical overload, and this helps to calm inflammation, nourish your skin and prevent (or reduce) food intolerances and allergies.

I have not discussed the science behind chemical intolerance in great detail here as I have covered this at length in my previous books. Your time is important so I feel it is more useful to give you the *best foods to eat* and the *best skin care ingredients* and the recipes to cook so you can FEEL and SEE how your skin responds. Wellness is an experiential thing.

Using the book

This book is divided into four sections.

'Part 1: The Healthy Skin Kitchen' covers evidence-based foods and nutrients for creating healthy skin plus effective ways to improve your gut microbiome and beat stress for life.

'Part 2: Skin care' covers the best topical skin care ingredients for glowing good skin and I have included a lush Oat and Zinc Bath Bomb recipe for you to try.

'Part 3: Signs, symptoms and solutions' — I realize many of you want specific advice on your skin problem/s so I have included a comprehensive table where you can look up your specific skin disorder (or related health problem) and find specific treatments. The topics covered are:

- » acne and pimples (p. 80)
- » alopecia (hair loss) (p. 80)
- » candidiasis (p. 81)
- » cellulite and cellulitis (p. 81)
- » chronic inflammatory response syndrome (CIRS; incl. mould sickness) (p. 82)
- » dandruff (p. 82)
- » dermatitis (p. 83)
- » eczema and dermatitis (all types, p. 84)
- » hidradenitis suppurativa (p. 84)
- » histamine/amine intolerance (p. 85)
- » hives/urticaria (p. 85)
- » keratosis pilaris (p. 85)
- » leaky gut (p. 86)
- » light sensitivity, photophobia (p. 86)
- » mast cell activation syndrome (p. 87)
- » pigmentation and age spots/liver spots (p. 87)
- » psoriasis (p. 87)
- » red skin syndrome (p. 88)
- » rosacea (p. 89)
- » salicylate sensitivity (p. 89)
- » wrinkles (p. 89)

'Part 4: Menus and recipes' is where you can find what to eat for your skin type. Not everyone can (or should) eat exactly the same foods. For example, a person with acne should not cook with the same oils as someone with dry skin or eczema. Refer to Chapter 7, 'Helpful guidelines' (p. 91) for information on choosing the best cooking oil and plant-based milks for your specific skin type.

I have divided the advice into six menus:

- » Menu 1: Clear skin (p. 97) for acne and oily skin types.
- » Menu 2: Firm and tone (p. 98) is the anti-ageing menu for cellulite, age spots and wrinkles.
- » Menu 3: Nourish/detox (p. 99) is for anyone who wants to support liver detoxification while nourishing their skin. It's also suitable for people with general

eczema, red skin syndrome and psoriasis.

» Menu 4: Low histamine/salicylate (p. 100) is a meal plan for people with severe eczema, psoriasis, rosacea and other types of chronic skin inflammation, who need a low salicylate/low histamine diet to help them look and feel well. It is also suitable for people following the Food Intolerance Diagnosis (FID) Program, which is a diagnostic program from my book *The Eczema Detox*. Due to space restraints I am not covering the FID instructions again in this book so if you need to diagnose food intolerances (such as salicylate intolerance) grab a copy of *The Eczema Detox*.

» Menu 5: Vegan (p. 102).

» Menu 6: Paleo/immune wellness (p. 103).

If you already have pretty good skin and you just want to maintain or improve it then you can eat any recipe in this book and choose whichever menus you like.

If you have red skin syndrome or a severe and chronic skin problem of any kind, please give yourself time and patience (and lots of kindness) and stay in touch with your doctor along the way.

> **Special notes**
>
> · If you have an allergy or intolerance to a specific food found in any of the recipes then simply avoid that food and find a suitable alternative.
>
> · If you have any medical problems or are taking medications, please chat with your doctor, psychologist or specialist before changing your diet or taking supplements.
>
> · My wish is to make your life easier so I briefly mention my supplements and skin care (plus other products and brands that are not my own) so you don't have to search hard for anything. You can, of course, choose to not use them.

How long will it take?

Normal, healthy skin renews itself every 28 days so if you have normal skin or mild skin problems I suggest following the diet for at least six weeks and then incorporate what you have learnt into your daily life. Try to be strict for six weeks so you can see the full effects and do not combine it with other natural treatments (such as herbs, as they are rich in salicylates) as this may affect your results. Some of my patients with chronic or severe eczema follow the program for years for continued relief, while others can expand their diet over time. Your skin will tell you how much time you need.

From my heart to yours

If you are struggling right now, take heart — you can create great skin from the inside out. And you can start today by feeding your skin better building materials (like the foods in Chapter 5) because you build your body with your knife and fork.

I hope you enjoy this cooking adventure, which is dotted with my favourite food photos, taken on my Canon 6D Mark II. The family photo (opposite) was taken by my talented friend Lyn McCreanor from In All Things Beautiful. Like a warm hug, I hope our images brighten your day too.

From my heart to yours, I wish you well on your journey to healthy skin and wellness. I'm right here with you via this book and I have experienced nutritionists working with me (at my office) who can be contacted via www.healthyskinkitchen.com if you need assistance and support along the way.

Love, health and happiness,

Karen Fischer xx

Your purchase helps children

This is my seventh and possibly my final health book so I wanted to do something special. So I am donating my *Healthy Skin Kitchen* royalty payments to the wonderful children's charity Save the Children (www.savethechildren.org.au). Your purchase will help to educate, support and feed children in Indigenous and disadvantaged communities, so thank you for buying this book. For details about the various children's programs we are helping to fund — there are so many heartwarming programs to choose from! — see www.healthyskinkitchen.com and sign up to our newsletter.

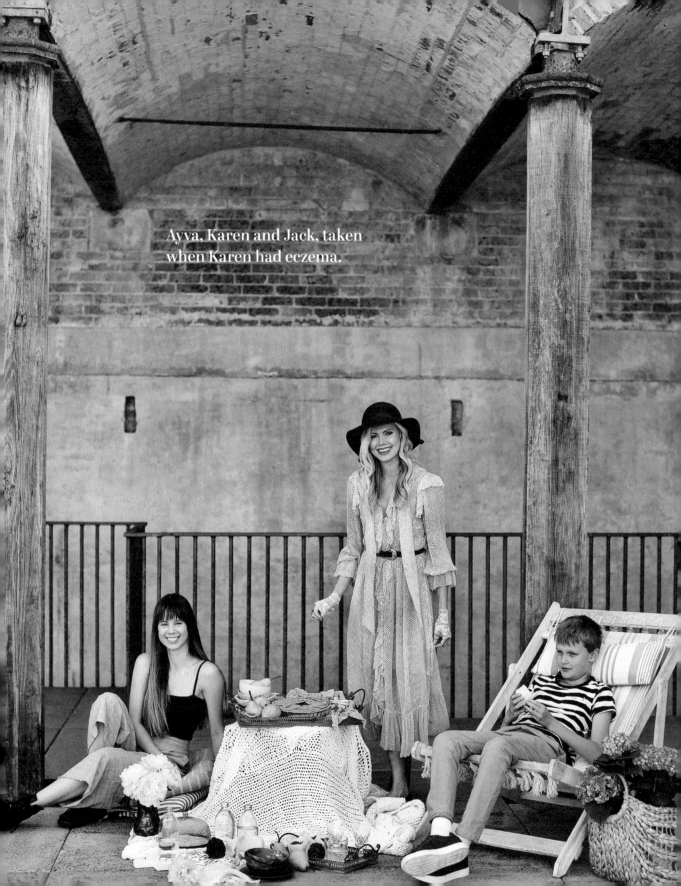

Ayva, Karen and Jack, taken
when Karen had eczema.

PART 1
The Healthy Skin Kitchen

Asparagus and Black Bean Soft Tacos (p. 155)

I want to talk about the path to wellness. Your skin is your largest organ — the one that keeps your insides in — and we need to treat it holistically (as a whole). What I mean by holistic is this: liver health is important for creating healthy skin but it's not the only governing factor. Gut health is also essential for glowing skin but you are more than just a long row of gastrointestinal tract. Even your thoughts and emotions (and eating while stressed or while watching the news) can affect your skin's appearance, so we should probably pay attention to this too. Your skin is a reflection of what is happening inside you. Part 1 of this book highlights effective ways to nourish your skin, your body and your mind in a new holistic way — encompassing the whole you — so your healthy inner life can be reflected outwards in the form of healthy looking skin.

Q: 'Do I need to follow every piece of advice or can I just make the recipes?'

Yes, make the recipes. As your skin is literally made from the foods you eat, I recommend everyone incorporate many of the recipes and foods in this book into their everyday life. I want to keep the HSK program simple (and do-able) so the following two chapters have information that is optional. These chapters outline some of the most exciting health research I have found, which helped me to change my body and create glowing, healthy skin, so I had to share this with you. But please pick the information that resonates with you. For example, if you have gut issues or sugar cravings, you might choose to follow the advice in Chapter 1, 'Constant cravings'. If you have autoimmune disorder, anxiety, depression or multiple food intolerances and allergies, the vagus nerve information could change your life. Or you might simply need to drink more water (most of us do).

For the wellness warriors who want to try it all, follow one activity at a time over the course of a month. Just don't stress yourself in the process because self-love and nourishing your body *should feel amazing*.

Q: 'I have mental health issues and stress is a major trigger of my skin problem. Is there advice in this book that can help me?'

Absolutely ... but I want to stress that I am not a psychologist or a psychotherapist: my advice regarding mental health is from my personal experience with anxiety and depression (which has now resolved) and from twenty years of working with patients with severe skin issues, which have often been triggered by stress and anxiety. I feel mental health is such an important part of skin wellness that it has to be at least briefly covered in this book. But your mental health is ultimately your responsibility. For me personally, mental health comes from letting go of the past, eating a nourishing diet, by being grateful, by 'growing the good' and from bravely living a life that feels authentic to me. This book can help you with the 'eating well' part so you can nourish your brain and body from the inside out.

Chapter 1

Constant cravings (it's not you, it's your microbiome)

As long as it's sweet your taste buds are on board, right? Can't finish your dinner without needing a dessert to top it off (even if you were full 5 minutes ago)? Whether it's treating yourself with home-brand chocolate or some fancy organic date latte, you could be a sugar addict and it's probably sabotaging your health and beauty goals. But now you can say it's not entirely your fault ... because your gut microbiome residents have a major say in what you crave.

What is your microbiome?

The ecosystem in your large intestine is called the microbiome and it consists of thousands of types of gut bacteria and fungi, both good and potentially pathogenic. Most of them are not invaders to be exterminated; they are beneficial colonizers that help to train your immune system, digest your food, protect against disease and produce some vitamins for good health including vitamin B12, thiamine (vitamin B1), riboflavin (vitamin B2) and vitamin K.

Your microbiome is fed by your diet: some microbes like chocolate, others crave broccoli and leafy greens. So what you eat determines who proliferates (and who dies) in your gut.

You might not be a choc-aholic after all

In one study, researchers noted that people who love chocolate have different microbial metabolites in their urine than people who feel indifferent to chocolate, despite eating identical amounts of chocolate during the study.[1] Scientists found that gut microbes can manipulate a person's eating behaviour, sometimes at the expense of the host's health (that's you), and they concluded that changing a person's gut microbiota leads to a change in cravings.[2]

According to researchers, our gut microbes can:

» generate cravings that suppress their competitors' growth (and maximize their own)
» induce a state of unease until you eat something that promotes their growth (hello chocolate cravings)
» produce toxins that alter your mood
» change taste receptors (seriously!)

» manipulate reward pathways (altering opioid/feel-good receptors in the gut)
» activate pain receptors.

And they do this by hijacking the *vagus nerve* which is the link between the gut and the brain.[3] Your vagus nerve is important for triggering feelings of being relaxed, calm and satisfied and it helps us to rest, digest and de-stress. So it's important to have control of this important nerve. (More on how to tone your vagus nerve on p. 18.)

Pathogenic yeasts such as Candida albicans make you crave sugar but when they are fed sugar they proliferate. This can trigger thrush and other yeast infection symptoms that can make you feel itchy, irritable and tired. Candidiasis treatments are covered on p. 81.

How to improve your gut microbiome (and kill cravings)

Your breakfast, lunch and dinner largely determine what types of gut bacteria and fungi thrive (or die) in your microbiome. For a healthier gut, feed your microbiome specific *prebiotic* foods. Don't get these mixed up with *probiotics* as they are not the same thing. Probiotics are supplements, and while beneficial, will do very little if your diet contains lots of sweet foods, sugar, alcohol and refined junk food. Prebiotics, on the other hand, are specific *fibre-rich* foods that literally feed your good bacteria so they thrive and crowd out the bad guys.

The good news is you can change your microbiome within three days of changing your diet. Your microbiome and gastrointestinal tract need at least 50 grams of fibre daily in order to be healthy. So load up with vegetables and other prebiotic foods to nourish your microbiome. Here are 12 prebiotic foods to feed beneficial microbes (and suppress the bad guys) in your microbiome.

12 foods for a healthy microbiome

apples	garlic
asparagus	green banana flour (p. 48)
banana (p. 48)	leeks (p. 38)
beetroot (p. 35)	oats (p. 39)
cabbage (see red cabbage, p. 50)	snow peas (mangetout)
cashews	spring onion (shallots/scallions) (p. 45)

You will find plenty of *Healthy Skin Kitchen* recipes that utilize these ingredients in the second half of this book.

What damages your microbiome?

· Overuse of antibiotics (two courses in a row will do it)
· Some medical drugs
· Smoking
· Frequent alcohol consumption
· Sugar
· Sodas/soft drinks
· Fast foods/junk food
· White flour products (cakes, biscuits, doughnuts, white pasta etc.)

Luckily gut bacteria have a short life cycle so changing your diet works quickly to change your cravings. You can effectively harvest new, healthier gut bacteria in a matter of days and you usually don't need probiotic supplements to do this.

How to kill major sugar cravings

I'm going to tell it to you straight ... The first thing you can do to kill sugar cravings is to cut off your gut microbiome's sugar supply. You do this by throwing away (or giving away) any sweet junk food you have in your home or office. Empty the sugar bowl and stop stocking up on chocolate. You can't eat it if it's not handy. Like a favourite child that you love, also give yourself *loving boundaries* around eating sweets: such as 'Sweets on Sunday' or 'Treat day is Friday' or 'Wine-o-clock is Friday after work' (not every day after work). Alcohol is liquid sugar. Obviously you can enjoy a treat when you are out with friends or family, but that's for special occasions, right?

The next section also contains more tips on killing cravings.

Fasting for highs and health

I felt a profound shift in my cravings and gut health after completing a short fast. Here is why fasting is an optional part of the Healthy Skin Kitchen ...

Fasting is choosing to abstain from eating food for a short period of time — usually for spiritual or health reasons. Fasting is not new. The ancient Egyptians, ancient Greeks and ancient Indians all did it and the Bible and other religious texts recommend it. Hippocrates (460–375 BC), known as the father of medicine, said fasting was a 'medical must' and 'excess food is against nature'. Now fasting is finally getting the scientific tick of approval in the area of beauty, immune system health, weight loss, disease management and longevity.[4] In fact, fasting can help to reduce obesity, asthma, high blood pressure, eczema, rheumatoid arthritis and premature ageing, to name a few.[5] Fasting also increases mental clarity and cuts cravings off at the knees as it profoundly changes your microbiome.

What type of fasts are best?

There are many different types of fasts but I prefer water fasting for short periods of time.

While longer fasts can be beneficial, they should be supervised by a health professional who is knowledgeable on fasting.

I also do not recommend fasts where you guzzle coffee, juice or teas during the fast as they miss the point of fasting, which is to *rest and repair the digestive system*. Drinking coffee and tea can irritate the stomach lining and worsen leaky gut, and fruit juices (no matter how freshly squeezed) can feed pathogenic microbes, play havoc with your blood sugar levels and spike insulin levels. And research backs this up. Scientists have repeatedly demonstrated how water fasting can change a person's microbiome for the better. One research project demonstrated how water fasting significantly reduced Fusobacterium in the microbiome (the bacteria that increases the risk of colon cancer) but a juice-only fast had no positive effect on Fusobacterium levels.[6]

1. Water fasting

A 36-hour water fast changed my life. Thirty-six hours was enough time to revive taste buds, kill cravings, rest the digestive system and begin the gut healing process, without feeling too hungry or deprived. Some tips and instructions are coming up shortly. You will need to sip 3–4 litres (6–8 pt) of filtered or spring water throughout the day.

2. Intermittent fasting

If you can't go without food for a whole day, intermittent fasting is another option. You basically fast for 12–16 hours a day (most of this occurs at night when you are sleeping) and you have two or three meals and sip 3 litres (6 pt) of filtered or spring water during the day. Remember the goal is to *rest and reset your digestive system* during the fasting hours, but you can have sweetener-free

Quick tips for a healthy microbiome

· Skip the sugar
· Do a short fast (see p. 12)
· Soak your fruit and vegies before eating them

Soak your fruit and veg

Washing your fruits and vegetables with good old tap water kills bacteria and removes pesticide residues (if not eating organic produce). However, if you live in Bali or a country where tap water is contaminated, wash your produce with bottled water. Ideally before chopping, slicing and dicing, soak your fruit and vegies in a bowl of water for up to 5 minutes.

If you are not sensitive to vinegar (which naturally contains salicylates, amines and sulphites/sulfites), you can add a splash of apple cider vinegar into the soaking water for an additional cleansing effect.

coffee during the *non-fasting* period each day, if you need to. I prefer organic decaf coffee, as it's a better option for skin health.

The benefits of water fasting and intermittent fasting

There are many scientifically proven benefits to fasting. These include:

» increased life span (if done on a frequent basis)
» improved immune system (fasting triggers the immune system to produce new white blood cells)
» increased stress resistance
» improved digestive system health (fasting allows it to clean and repair itself)
» more sensitive taste buds (bland food is suddenly bursting with flavour so you don't rely on sugar-laden sauces)
» reduced/relieved candidiasis (Candida albicans infestation)
» improved gut microbiome
» damaged cells are killed
» reduced inflammation in the body
» decreased blood glucose and insulin
» increased stress resistance in the brain
» reduced blood pressure
» reduced body fat
» improvement in concentration and alertness.[7]

Who should not fast?

Ultimately it is up to you, the individual, to determine if a mini fast or intermittent fasting is right for you and your health situation. Medical or family supervision during a fast is recommended. If you have red skin syndrome or heart disease or are frail, very sick, underweight, pregnant, breastfeeding, a child or taking medications, skip fasting and focus on other activities in this book.

My first fasting experience changed my life

I initially did a 36-hour fast because I was covered in eczema and everything I ate made me itchy, so I thought a day of *not eating* might give me some relief. I was desperate. So I ate a nice big dinner topped with Caramelized Leek Sauce (which was sweet) at about 7 p.m., took a magnesium and calcium supplement, watched some TV and then went to bed. The next day I didn't eat anything and I sipped about 4 litres (8 pt) of spring water (natural, non-carbonated) throughout the day. Then I went to bed that night feeling hungry. Boy was I hungry. But I survived.

The next day at 7 a.m. I drank a small smoothie for breakfast to gently reintroduce foods into my well-rested digestive tract (The Blue Healer, p. 112). My tastebuds now picked up flavours like they had never done before. Lunch tasted great, without salt or any sauce or other flavouring. And I could no longer enjoy sweet foods, like the Caramelized Leek Sauce I ate two days before — it suddenly seemed far too sweet and I could not eat it with dinner. Had to throw it out. In fact, I could not stand to eat anything sweet for several months.

But I was in savoury heaven as all other foods tasted fantastic ... Chicken and plain vegetables were suddenly bursting with flavours that were sweet and salty and tangy all at the same time (seriously), *with absolutely no seasoning or salt or oil*. And since my fast I no longer need to add any sauce to the healthy foods I cook in order to love them. I still occasionally use homemade dips and sauces on my meals when shooting them for this book, and I have included sauces and dips in my recipes for those of you who have not reset your taste buds.

After the fast, each day I found it so easy to pile my dinner plate high with vegies (alongside protein and maybe a flatbread or two) and it was easy to skip dessert. Four months later my body was completely cellulite-free and rash-free thanks to my new way of eating, which I am sharing with you in this book. It all began with a one-day fast.

How to begin your fast

1. CHOOSE YOUR DAY OFF

I suggest doing your fast on a day when you can relax or work from home. You might feel a little tired and low in energy but you can exercise, do yoga or meditate while fasting if you want to. You will probably feel hungry so keep your water bottle handy and distract yourself with a good book, a nanna nap, a relaxing hobby and/or Netflix. While I fasted I sat at my computer and banged out a couple of blog posts — my concentration was amazing as my body was not busy digesting food.

2. CHOOSE YOUR TIME LIMIT — 24 HOURS OR 36 HOURS OF FASTING

So you have picked a day. Now you need to work out how long you can (or want to) go without food:

» A 24-hour fast means you never miss dinner (you just skip one breakfast and one lunch). For example, you finish eating dinner around 7 p.m. on Day 1, then you eat dinner on Day 2 at 7 p.m. (and sip water in between).

» A 36-hour fast means you will miss breakfast, lunch and dinner on one day. So you will go to bed hungry for one night only. You can sip water throughout the day and this helps you to feel full(ish).

You will need to carefully choose your first meal that breaks the fast, as you don't want to eat too much or eat something that is sweet (your gut is now like a baby's — the first thing you eat gives a specific gut bacteria a head start, so don't feed the choc-aholics or sugar fiends). Feed the vegie lovers first, with vegies (of course).

A 36-hour fast worked for me but if you have any health problems, please seek the advice of a fasting expert before doing a fast for any length of time, or skip this optional step.

Fasting tips

» If in doubt, get a medical check-up to see if you are well enough to do a fast.

» One-day fasts are safe but I still suggest having someone at home or who can visit you to intermittently supervise your fast.

» Ensure you are not malnourished. Take a magnesium supplement (p. 58) and a multivitamin formula for a few days beforehand so your body is topped up with vitamins and minerals.

» Before you begin, spend a week using up the food in your refrigerator (and don't restock it). Plan your breaking-the-fast meal so it's ready to go when you're done. Tip: you will be less tempted if there are no decadent or sweet foods within reach.

» Put a note inside (or outside) your refrigerator and pantry reminding you that it is FAST DAY, just in case you forget.

» During your fast it's important to drink about 3–4 litres (6–8 pt) of water, sipped throughout the day. However, drink less than 1 litre (2 pt) per hour as you don't want to stress your kidneys by guzzling too quickly.

» Don't complain or whinge as this only makes it harder to achieve your goals — it can lead to self-sabotage and make you unpleasant to be around.

» That hunger pain you are feeling is the gut doing a clean up — it's sweeping the floor and putting out the garbage so don't interrupt it!

» If you feel really unwell, stop the fast, eat a light snack and seek advice — your health is your responsibility, so if it feels wrong for you, don't fast.

Best meals to break your fast

It's important to choose a light meal (or have a smaller serving) for your first meal after a fast. Do not add any sweetener or salt during cooking — you can add a tiny bit of salt after eating a few mouthfuls, *if the meal really needs salt*. Pick one meal and buy the ingredients so it's easy to prepare after your fast:

Breakfasts to choose from (if doing a 36-hour fast):

» The Blue Healer (p. 112) or any other smoothie recipe (pp. 109–110)
» Cabbage Steaks with Beet Cream (p. 125)
» Sweet Potato Toast (p. 123) — the savoury options
» Green Detox Soup (p. 179).

Dinners to choose from (if doing a 24-hour fast):

» Beet Detox Soup (p. 149)
» Green Detox Soup (p. 179)
» Sweet Potato Boats (p. 180)
» Healthy Fish Tacos (p. 187) in lettuce leaf cups
» San Choy Bau (p. 159) in lettuce leaf cups, no vermicelli or flatbread.

Spend the last hour or two of your fast cooking a really nice meal to enjoy.

Chapter 2
Create an inner sanctuary (for your vagus nerve)

Just breathe out deeply. Might seem like shallow advice but this simple trick is rooted in some damn exciting science. Mindfully breathing in and (in particular) slowly breathing out stimulates the vagus nerve, which puts a brake on the stress response in your body. Even Harvard Medical School are on board, with an article in *Harvard Health Publishing* praising belly breathing for its ability to stimulate the vagus nerve to reduce stress and lower blood pressure.[1]

What is the vagus nerve and why should you care?

The vagus nerve is the longest nerve in your body. It has two main branches that run down either side of your spine and they connect your brain to your organs including your gut, intestines, colon, liver, lungs and heart.[2] It's like a network of telephone wires that allows your brain to speak to your organs and vice versa. You've probably heard of the *gut–brain connection*, but we could also say *lung–brain connection* and *heart–brain connection* as many of your organs converse with your brain via the vagus nerve.[3] Vagus nerve wellness is vital for your mental wellbeing and organ health but it can be damaged by alcoholism, psychological trauma and diabetes.[4] The good news is, this communication superhighway can be monitored, stimulated and improved, as I'll discuss shortly.

Vagal tone: put a brake on your stress

The activity of the vagus nerve is referred to as vagal tone. High vagal tone is linked to good health and low vagal tone is associated with various health problems. Like a tranquilizer to calm you down, vagal tone refers to how well your vagus nerve recovers from stress.[5] When the vagus nerve is stimulated, a range of calming and soothing neurotransmitters, such as acetylcholine, are released and your body relaxes. And it's not just relaxing: vagus nerve stimulation activates regions in the brain to relieve pain and inhibit inflammation in the body.[6] High vagal tone can also make your voice sound more resonant, relaxed and deep as the vagus nerve is attached to your voice box. It makes sense that tense people sound tense when they speak. You might even stutter or stumble over your words when vagal tone is poor.

The mind–skin connection

It's not just your voice that sufferers when vagal tone is suppressed: poor vagal tone can lead to various skin disorders. Here's why.

It is well established that stress can trigger all sorts of skin problems. You might have experienced this first-hand during stressful situations like a first date (hello stress pimple). And it is common knowledge that psychological stress can trigger eczema.[7] While stress is not the only trigger of skin disorders such as eczema, it is an important factor that is often overlooked in favour of short-term band-aid solutions. Researchers have found that psychological stress impairs skin barrier function, which is often seen in people with eczema and dry skin, and stress reduces immune function in the epidermis layer of the skin.[8]

» Researchers found that stress during pregnancy increases the risk of childhood eczema.[9]
» Children with atopic eczema are more likely to have ADHD-like behaviour because of a reduced HPA axis response to stress.[10] This is a sign of poor vagal tone in children with eczema as the vagus nerve stimulates the hypothalamic–pituitary–adrenal (HPA) axis, which then regulates the stress response.[11]

So it's important that we address our stress levels if we want to create healthy skin, right? Over the years I have worked with hundreds of patients who reported that stress was the initial trigger of their skin disease. We talk about the detrimental effects of stress as if it is beyond our control. I am guilty of this too. I suffered from work stress yet I failed to take time off when I could have implemented strategies to give my body what it needed to rest, restore and revive. But I didn't know how. 'Stress' seems so foreign and out of our control. But it's not … Now we can all do something to counteract stress because *vagus nerve research* gives us a scientific road map to follow, and it's measurable too.

Knowing about the vagus nerve and how to monitor vagal tone is a wonderful way to teach yourself to be more resilient to stress and ultimately more relaxed, calm and confident. It does not mean that suddenly stress will not exist in your life — there will still be bad traffic, thoughtless people and work demands — but your body will simply handle life's stressors better and you will *feel* better on the inside. Nor will you become more naive or bury your head in the sand in some phony utopian dream … The aim is to gently learn to manage life better with tools that science has proven effective. The saying 'Keep calm and carry on' sums up vagal tone nicely.

Why improve vagal tone for stress relief? Can't you just give me a pill or a potion?

Let me start by saying if you need to take medications, please keep taking them. You can work with your therapist or doctor *and* take steps to improve your vagal tone — it's not an all-or-nothing scenario here. But know this: improving your vagal tone not only helps you to calm down and de-stress, it floods your body with feel-good chemicals and *anti-inflammatory* chemicals, which can help to combat inflammation and pain in the body.[12] So if you want to feel good, read on. Vagal tone is the key here as it halts the stress response, like flicking on a light switch: you just need to know how to stimulate it, and I'll discuss how shortly.

How vagally toned are you?

People are born with various degrees of vagal tone — some infants naturally have high vagal tone, while others have poorer tone.[13] Researchers found that infants who cry more usually have poorer vagal tone.[14] And while a person's level of vagal tone can remain constant for months or years, vagal tone can be damaged or suppressed by psychological trauma and other life events — and this can lead to a predisposition for illness. On the other hand, vagal tone can also be improved with mindfulness and relaxation techniques.[15] So the good news is you have the power to change your vagal inheritance.

Poor vagal tone is associated with:

- » histamine-induced itchy skin (pruritus)[16]
- » atopic dermatitis/eczema[17]
- » food allergies[18]
- » irritable bowel disease and IBS[19]
- » increased intestinal permeability (leaky gut)[20]
- » sensitivity to stress[21]
- » post-traumatic stress disorder[22]
- » heightened emotional reactivity[23]
- » psychological problems in children and teenagers[24]
- » anxiety disorders[25]
- » depression[26]
- » panic disorders[27]
- » bipolar disorder[28]
- » stuttering[29]
- » Tourette syndrome[30]
- » epilepsy[31]
- » inflammation.[32]

Inflammation, allergies and the vagus nerve

Your immune system is designed to protect your body from invasion but it can also attack you if it is unhealthy. Your skin acts as a barrier to keep out the germs and other bad guys, and this is called innate immunity. According to research, TH1/TH2 immune system imbalance can occur in people with eczema and allergic diseases, where TH1 immunity is excessively low and TH2 immunity is predominant, resulting in immune system dysfunction.[33] Now researchers have linked TH1/TH2 balance with the vagus nerve, which has anti-inflammatory properties that affect the gut's immune system and TH1/TH2 balance.[34] The researchers from Belgium demonstrated that vagus nerve stimulation significantly decreased inflammation in animals with allergies, and the researchers suggested that vagus nerve stimulation could be beneficial in treating food allergies and other immune-related diseases.[35]

How to test your cardiac vagal tone

The good news is you can test your *cardiac vagal tone* to gauge how good your vagal tone really is. Heart rate variability (HRV) testing is a simple medical test conducted by doctors and heart specialists, where the measurement of time between each heartbeat is recorded. It's an easy way to identify nervous system imbalance. How HRV works is the vagus nerve 'listens' to your breathing rate via lung stretch receptors and it adapts your heart rate in response. A higher (and healthier) vagal tone is associated with *higher* heart rate variability (HRV).

According to Harvard Health Publishing, medical doctors and heart specialists perform this simple test using an electrocardiogram but there are also apps (such as Elite HRV) and heart rate monitors that you can use at home. It's analyzing the results that can get a bit tricky, which is why consulting with your doctor can be helpful. An app could be a good way to create initial self-awareness, but after delving into vagal tone exercises for quite some time, I can tell you that in my experience *you know* when your vagal tone is high as you feel so damn good: you feel calmer and annoyances such as bad traffic, bank queues and pandemics don't excessively bother you; your skin stops itching (if applicable), and you generally feel happy, for no particular reason.

The good news is, you are totally responsible for your vagal tone — it can be manipulated and improved at any time — and it's an ongoing process that can make you feel good almost instantly once you get the hang of it. I have created an activity chart for you to get more vagally toned within 30 days (see p. 26).

Activities that increase vagal tone

» Deep and slow breathing (see p. 26)[36]
» Meditation such as body scan meditation and transcendental meditation[37]
» Yoga and chanting[38] (for online yoga and meditation classes, see 'Helpful resources', p. 198)
» Exercise
» Massage: there are pressure points near the base of your spine, ears, shoulders and clavicles that activate the vagus nerve and help you to relax
» Listening to relaxing music where the music beat is slower than a heartbeat
» Singing and voice training exercises
» Gargling salt water: it exercises the larynx and stimulates the nuclei of the brain stem and parasympathetic (rest and digest) nervous system
» Take a cold shower or splash your face with cold water
» Get grounded. Research on preterm infants revealed that exposure to electromagnetic fields (caused by incubators) can adversely affect vagal tone but when the infants were electrically grounded to the earth (also known as 'earthing'), their vagal tone improved by 67 per cent and their skin voltage dropped by 95 per cent.[39] Earthing is where you spend time in nature and touch the ground with your bare feet. If going outdoors is not possible (i.e. during winter), you can buy earthing products such as an earthing sheet to sleep on at night or an earthing mat to put under your computer's keyboard and mouse.

You can't have relaxed nerves if you feel anxious, unloved or lonely. The antidote is gratitude — it sends your body 'safety cues' via the vagus nerve to create a deep sense of calm and connectedness.

The great exhale: vagal tone breathing exercise

Vagal tone is highest when you are exhaling, and a longer exhale triggers the rest and digest part of the nervous system. You can do this type of breathing anywhere, you don't have to lie down (but it's great before sleep), you could be on a train, on a plane, at work or sitting in a beanbag. Just do it as often as you can, especially when you are feeling stressed, anxious, sad, rushed or entrenched in mind chatter. Ensure your posture is good and ideally do the breathing exercises before each meal to flip on your 'digest' switch, and again before bed to flick on your 'rest' switch to help you sleep.

It's easy: you just need to double the length of your exhale.

Next level vagal tone exercises

We have discussed some good standard vagal tone activities that are recommended by doctors and wellness gurus alike. Quite frankly, though, you can chant and breathe deeply all day long but if you feel lonely, anxious or unsafe (whether real or imagined), you will probably have poor vagal tone. You might be 'doing everything right' but if you feel stressed or are constantly whingeing about your life and the people in it, you are slowly shutting down your vagus nerve. This affects every organ from your skin, heart and gut to your lungs and brain (and your mental wellbeing).

Let's be frank: you might need to move to a safer neighbourhood, leave an abusive partner or forgive the past, but if that's not possible (just yet) there are 'next level' exercises you can do to calm your mind and promote vagal tone while you get your life together. You don't have to move to Beverly Hills or meet the perfect partner, *just focus on compassion and gratitude* — they're free and available to you right now. And these exercises are suitable for all ages: even young children can benefit from them.

Good vagal tone is an attitude of gratitude

The vagus nerve is the nerve of compassion.[40] Psychologists have found that children with good vagus nerve activity are more cooperative and giving.[41] And people with high vagal tone are more prone to feeling gratitude, compassion, love and happiness.[42] It also works in reverse: *you can do activities that focus on gratitude and compassion to stimulate and improve your vagus nerve.*

Your vagal tone is peaking when you get that 'warm fuzzy' feeling inside and you can create this feeling any time you like — it just takes practice. It also works well to relieve some types of pain, reduce inflammation and stop a bone-deep itch in its tracks (trust me, it works). Vagal tone feels good as it floods your bloodstream with natural painkillers and other feel-good chemicals. And if you need statistical evidence, you can monitor your HRV at the same time, with fancy apps and a heart rate monitor.

Here are some 'next level' vagal tone exercises that have been scientifically proven to stimulate the vagus nerve.

> **Vagal tone breathing exercise**
>
> Breathe in for three counts and then breathe out for a count of six. Relax your body and feel your breath move down towards your belly as you breathe in. Be present. Simply count in your head. Do this at least five times. Then as you improve, lengthen your breaths: breathe in for four counts and then breathe out for eight counts, and so on.

1. Socially connect with others (in your head!)

Do you have a friend who is happy and laughs a lot? Call them. Laughing with friends and family triggers the release of 'feel-good' chemicals and it lowers the stress response in your body. You don't even need to be with them in person ... Just thinking about (and picturing in your mind) the cracking good time you had with them stimulates your vagus nerve. The more you think about (and savour) the good times, the better you feel. Let me repeat that — you do not need to actually be in the same room as the friend/lover/family member in order to feel socially connected and loved — you can just use your imagination to get a warm fuzzy feeling flowing through your body. It's called 'savouring the good', according to neuropsychologist Dr Rick Hanson, author of the brilliant book *Hardwiring Happiness*. And it helps to rewire your brain to feel happier if done frequently and with mindfulness.

Why does this work? Because your brain cannot tell the difference between what is real and what is imagined.[43] It's a big statement but it's true ... For example, researchers scanned the brains of people as they played the piano and compared them to people who only *imagined* they were playing the piano (and there was a comparison group who did neither). The results confirmed that the piano players and the people who imagined playing the piano had the same brain scan results.[44] That's why you are better off watching *Friends* (or another light comedy) rather than a horror film or thriller — because your brain cannot tell what is real or imagined and it feels stressed when watching stressful events on TV. And if you tell yourself you are lonely and you dwell on the times you were rejected, your vagal tone becomes poorer and poorer.

2. Laugh more, bitch less

Your brain and body feel good when watching something funny, as laughter triggers a 'safety signal' to the rest of your body via the vagus nerve. How brilliant is that? Laughing promotes higher vagal tone and it produces feelings of social connectedness.[45] So instead of bitching about your life or watching the nightly news, flick on a Netflix comedy special and laugh your way to good vagal health.

3. Gratitude therapy

A study by the National Institute of Health found that gratitude triggers the brain's hypothalamus, which is the centre that controls stress and sleep, to release the 'reward' neurotransmitter dopamine which makes you feel good.[46] So gratitude can literally make you feel better.

During the COVID-19 pandemic in 2020, after moments of panic, I practised gratitude in order to stay calm, happy and well. My friends and I sent funny memes and videos to each other. We laughed a lot while being separated. I was grateful to be well, grateful my family and friends were well and I knew the pandemic would end and life might somehow be better after it. I was grateful for less traffic, reduced pollution and improved sanitation (my son finally learnt to wash his hands properly!). While some people did panic, in Australia we also saw kindness everywhere: landlords, the government and even banks helped people who could not pay their rent or mortgages during lockdown. While many people lost their jobs and incomes, some took this opportunity to start new online businesses and managed to thrive. Others enjoyed some much-needed time off to rest and relax.

Trauma researcher Dr Stephen Porges from Indiana University says that practising gratitude can help to condition your vagus nerve, giving 'safety cues' to your nervous system.[47] So whatever you can do to *feel safe* will help your nervous system and improve vagal tone. I must admit at times I did feel unsafe during the pandemic, but it was usually after watching the statistics on the news. It took time to talk my nervous system down off the ledge, but having 'an attitude of gratitude' really did help.

Q: 'How do I know vagal toning is working for me?'

Here is my personal story to illustrate the changes that can occur. Growing up I was very shy, I had a mild stutter and a lazy tongue that made me mispronounce my words occasionally. It was not bad enough to need therapy and in my twenties I improved my speech by doing voice-training lessons. The voice exercises enabled me to work on-air in television but if I stopped the voice training (or if I felt socially isolated or rejected), my voice would become weak and I would slightly stutter and mispronounce the odd word once again. These were all signs of low vagal tone, which should have been investigated years ago. Voice training was really a band-aid solution for me – anxiety (which I thought was just shyness) and feeling unsafe were the underlying conditions that affected my nervous system.

Then a bout of stress in my forties caused my vagus nerve to shut down and I experienced heart palpitations, sudden weight loss, insomnia and head-to-toe skin inflammation (my immune system basically went psycho). I was a strong person on the outside – I did a great job at looking after myself and my children, I was successful at work and had lots of friends – but I was overly sensitive on the inside, a work-aholic and I had stopped having fun a long time ago.

Along with tweaking my diet (which cleared up half of my skin problem in a matter of days), I delved deeply into waking up my vagus nerve. Within six months I went from feeling stressed and anxious to feeling calm and sleeping soundly, and the last patches of my skin rash cleared up. What surprised me most was the dramatic change in my voice, which happened within a few months – this occurred because the vagus nerve is attached to the voice box. My voice became more resonant and now has a lovely tone (when I am super relaxed it is almost husky and deep). And I don't need to do voice training anymore; I speak clearly and pronounce my words perfectly, *because I finally feel safe* as gratitude and laughing sends 'safety cues' to my body.

A calm body heals better than a stressed one.

Your personal journey to wellness might manifest in different ways to my own. But researchers did find that vagus nerve stimulation (to treat patients with epilepsy) can dramatically change a person's voice and improve speech in people who are going to speech therapy, so this is a common response, not just my own.

Q: 'That's a lot of info. What are some easy activities I can begin with?'

It really is all about creating an inner sanctuary where you feel calm, connected and safe. And that begins with your thoughts. Your brain, which is attached to your vagus nerve, governs your stress response. Ask yourself: what makes me feel connected and safe, without being co-dependent and needy? What makes me feel calm, without resorting to unhealthy vices? I have created a vagus nerve workout program for you … As mentioned, I am not a psychologist, but personally I'm a vagal tone convert. Most of these activities only take a few minutes at a time, some only fifteen seconds. Set yourself a 30-day challenge as this will help you make vagal toning a habit that becomes second nature.

Vagus nerve workout — 30-day challenge

Do the following activities daily. You can do them all or one each day but the more often you do them, the better your vagal tone will be. It changed my life.

Morning vagal toning	Midday vagal toning	Vagal in the evening
Time: less than 1 minute Wake up and say thank you: before you step out of bed think about three things you are grateful for, smile and dwell on them for a moment. Then get out of bed and smile at yourself in the mirror – it sends the body natural painkillers and 'feel-good' chemicals, so just do it.	**Time: less than 1 minute** While working at your desk (or wherever) take a deep, slow breath in, and a longer exhale: breathe in for a count of 3, out for 6, then in for 4, out for 8. If you are sitting at a desk all day, take a quick break and go outside and walk barefoot on the grass or touch a tree with your bare hands to ground your body.	**Time: at least 5 minutes** When you get home, meditate or do deep breathing exercises to help you disconnect from work and the busyness of the day. Or call a funny friend and chat: avoid complaining and focus on connecting and making each other laugh. Afterwards, take 15 seconds to savour (relive) the happy feelings and feel grateful for the friendship.

Morning vagal toning	Midday vagal toning	Vagal in the evening
Time: at least 15 seconds Have a cold shower (or end the shower with cold water) and say 'good morning vagus nerve!' (that bit is optional). Laugh for at least 15 seconds while showering: it will help you to cope with the cold.	**Time: 5 minutes** Savour the good: daydream about a meaningful conversation or event you had with a friend or loved one, until you feel connected, warm and fuzzy. Conjure feelings of safety and love – the people don't have to be around you to feel that deep connection, you just have to think about it and smile. Be grateful.	**Time: however long it takes to cook dinner** Play relaxing music while you cook dinner: I have created a 'Dancing in the Kitchen' playlist on Spotify for you to enjoy while you cook and eat healthy food (Spotify information can be found on p. 199).
Time: 15 minutes Breathe deeply and play relaxing music while you eat breakfast to flip on the 'rest and digest' switch (I have created a Vagus Nerve Wellness playlist for you on Spotify, see p. 199) or eat breakfast while sitting barefoot on the grass in your garden.	**Time: at least 30 minutes** Exercise at some point throughout the day, such as yoga (any activity will do) or if you are unable to exercise due to illness or limitations, sing and do the vagal tone breathing exercises (p. 23) (see online yoga classes in 'Helpful resources', p. 198).	**Time: at least 15 minutes** Play sleep music while getting ready for bed (and on low volume when you get into bed, if desired). I have created Sleep Well, a playlist on Spotify to flip your nervous system into 'rest' mode (see p. 199).
Time: less than 1 minute Heal yourself each day: smile at yourself in the mirror and say 'I love you' to the little child that still resides in you – send compassion and love to yourself (someone has to!). Say something nice to a family member or someone you live with. The good feeling a genuine compliment produces (for both you and the recipient) helps to rewire your brain to feel more calm, connected and safe.	**Time: less than 1 minute** Become aware of negative thinking: worry, disaster thinking, complaining about others (in your head or aloud) or criticizing and judging yourself. When you notice negative self-chatter *retrain and redirect your mind* with a pattern-breaking phrase such as: 'Stop', 'All is well' or 'It's okay' Redirect your mind and develop an attitude of gratitude.	**Time: less than 5 minutes** Weather permitting, before bed go outside and ground your body by touching a plant or the earth with your bare hands or feet. When you get into bed think about everything you are grateful for until you feel warm and fuzzy inside, then keep going and savour the good feelings. Be grateful for your life.

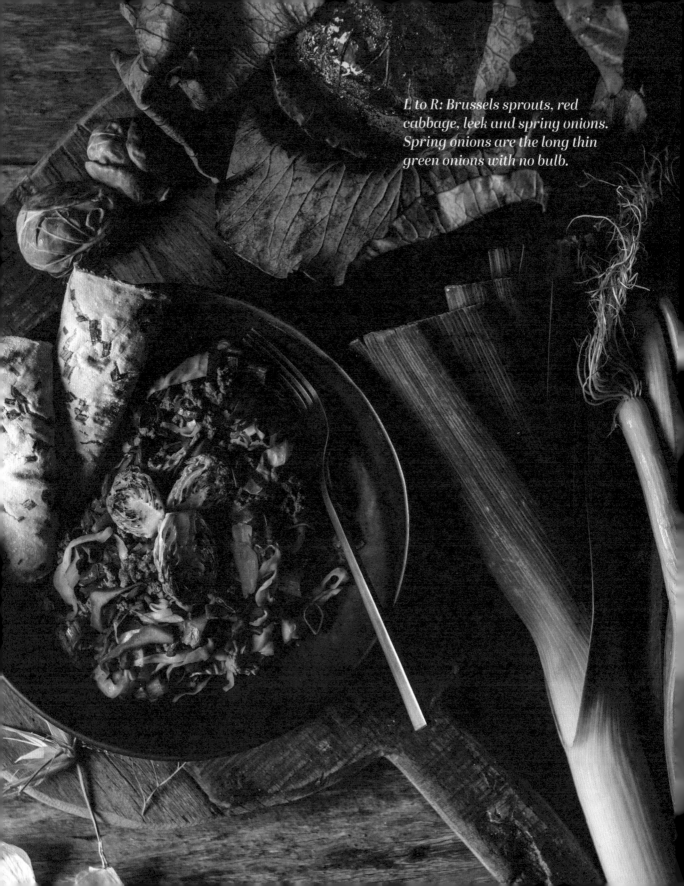

L to R: Brussels sprouts, red cabbage, leek and spring onions. Spring onions are the long thin green onions with no bulb.

Chapter 3
Eat this for beautiful skin

Your body is the home that you live in so why not treat it like the temple it truly is? After all, you can't exchange your body for a newer model if it suddenly breaks down or wears out. I often marvel at how some people are so focused on making money, meanwhile they eat crap and treat their body like a garbage tip. Seriously, if you have good health and great skin, you are super rich in my book. Trust me, if your skin itched from head to toe, you would know this is true. If your body constantly ached, you would know this is true. So I have hand-picked 17 fabulous skin-loving foods for you to try. You'll notice that most of them are not the typical superfoods, as many did not meet the criteria for this book. So I chose the top 17 foods based on the following criteria.

The top 17 healthy skin foods

All of these foods are:

1. Healthy and nutritious: they either contain powerful anti-inflammatory substances or they're fibre-rich prebiotics or they have alkalizing properties or they soothe and soften and hydrate your skin.
2. Low allergy: they do not contain common allergens.
3. Low chemical: they are classed as either low or moderate in salicylates, so they give your liver a little break from processing high levels of this chemical. For example, foods such as turmeric, tea and almonds are very rich in salicylates so they are not suitable for everyone — this book shows you low chemical alternatives that are delicious.
4. Low histamine: the top 17 do not contribute to high histamine levels in the body. Many trendy foods, such as fermented foods, are incredibly rich in histamines — chemicals produced by the body during an allergic response — so they are not right for everyone and do not feature in this book.
5. Lower GI: high GI foods excessively and repeatedly spike blood sugar, which increases the risk of type 2 diabetes, heart disease, obesity and acne. So the following foods are low GI (with the exception of beetroot) because healthy blood means healthy skin.
6. The top 17 are completely free of artificial additives.

Q: 'What is alkalizing?'

A healthy body has acid–alkaline balance, and the word 'alkalizing' is used to describe if a food is (or becomes) alkalizing within your body. You do not need to eat a diet consisting of 100 per cent alkalizing foods – your meals should be balanced – so you can eat acidifying foods such as meats, beans, grains and seafood, as long as you also eat vegetables. All vegetables are alkalizing in varying amounts, except for cooked spinach and cooked tomato which are acid-producing, and some fruits, such as banana, are alkalizing. Powerful/highly alkalizing foods are rare and include beetroot (beets) and all sprouts such as pea shoots and mung bean sprouts, which are included in the following list.

1. Pea shoots

Pea shoots are the lifesavers of the plant world. Here's why. Not only are pea shoots highly alkalizing and rich in histamine-lowering vitamin C, they're a super source of a potent anti-histamine enzyme called diamine oxidase, also referred to as DAO.[1] DAO plays a starring role in alleviating allergic reactions, anaphylaxis and histamine intolerance.[2] So it's an incredibly important enzyme that can unfortunately decline as you age.

A healthy body typically makes enough DAO, but it can get depleted if you frequently drink alcohol or caffeine or get too stressed. Caffeine from coffee, energy drinks and tea (including green tea and mate tea) interfere with the production of DAO in the body,[3] so if you are enjoying several cups daily it could lead to increased allergies and food intolerances. Some types of prescription drugs, including antibiotics and aspirin, block DAO production; and nutritional deficiencies in copper, vitamin B6, vitamin C and zinc cause DAO deficiency because they are required for DAO production.[4]

And when you eat a histamine-rich diet that includes seafood, nuts, fast foods, cheese, wine/alcohol, chocolate, and fermented foods and sauces, your body needs higher levels of DAO and other enzymes in order to cope with the influx of histamine. It's a fine balance between enjoying your food and allowing your body to make enough DAO (without blocking it).

Some bodies just can't cope due to ageing or illness and some of us aren't living the right lifestyle to support DAO production so we need a little extra help. If you have diagnosed histamine intolerance or allergies, animal-derived DAO supplements are available but they are expensive and come from animal sources so they are not an option for everyone. The good news is you can make your own natural plant DAO by sprouting peas and mung beans. You can also buy pea shoots (also called pea sprouts) at various supermarkets. You simply wash them and pop them into a smoothie as the blender's pulverizing action releases the DAO.

THE RESEARCH

» Low levels of the histamine-degrading enzymes DAO and MAO are found in people with eczema and atopic dermatitis.[5]

» Pea shoot DAO significantly protects the heart and lungs from anaphylaxis damage when subjects are injected with histamine and exposed to allergens.[6]

RECIPES

Make the DAO Smoothie (p. 109) or The Blue Healer smoothie (p. 112) and drink your DAO-rich smoothie with your main meals. Or sprinkle pea shoots on salads such as the Quinoa and Chicken Salad with Beet Cream (p. 163) and Sweet Potato Boats (p. 180).

STORAGE

» Store pea sprouts wrapped in a paper towel in a sealed container in the refrigerator — they will last seven to ten days if they are fresh.

» Always rinse them in water before serving.

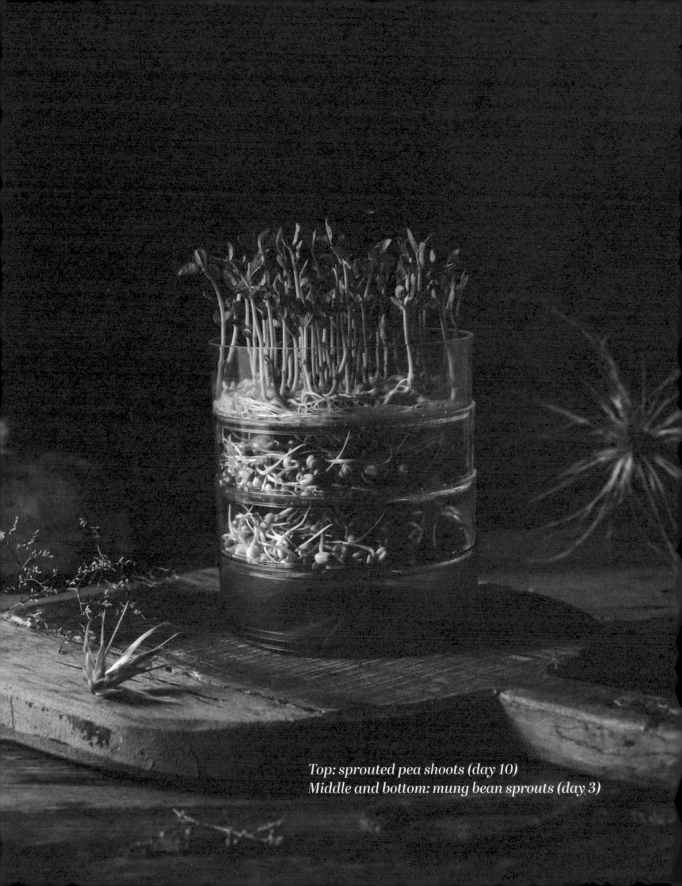

Top: sprouted pea shoots (day 10)
Middle and bottom: mung bean sprouts (day 3)

How to sprout pea shoots

Makes 1 batch, preparation time 10 minutes, takes 10–12 days to grow

You will need a seed sprouter (such as a three-tiered one) or a glass container, and netting or fine cheesecloth to cover.

- ⅓ cup dried peas (whole peas, not split)
- tap water

Rinse the dried peas and discard any discoloured or damaged ones. Split peas will not sprout so ensure they are whole. Place them into a seed sprouter (you can buy them from large hardware stores and online. I bought Mr Fothergill's Kitchen Seed Sprouter). Water them, allowing the water to drain away. Tip: in countries where the tap water is safe to drink, chlorinated tap water works best as it prevents them from going mouldy.

Place the sprouting container on a benchtop away from direct sunlight and cover with a net or cloth to keep any bugs out. Water the peas three times daily, draining away excess water, for 10–12 days (depending on the weather: if it's hot they sprout faster than in cold weather).

On day 9 or 10, place them in a dark cupboard for 1–2 days. Sprouts and seedlings produce more DAO when grown in the dark — the stress caused by lack of light makes them product more DAO as a protective response.[7]

When they are ready, trim the stems at the base, just above the pea. Store the shoots in the refrigerator in a sealed container (discard the pea and roots). Use within 10 days. Consume them raw with salads or, for better absorption of DAO, liberate the DAO enzyme by liquefying the seedlings in a smoothie and consume it with your main meals.[8]

2. Mung bean sprouts

Sprout your own superfood — it's easy. Mung bean sprouts are like little alkalizing bombs as they are one of the few strongly alkalizing foods you can add to your meals to create acid–alkaline balance. Mung bean sprouts are a natural source of DAO.[9] When mung beans are sprouted, the levels of vitamin C, DAO and quercetin dramatically increase — all have a histamine-lowering effect within the body and they help to reduce inflammation in the gastrointestinal tract.

Mung bean sprouts contain magnesium, vitamin K, folate and potassium and they are classed as low salicylate, making them ideal for people with skin inflammation.

RECIPES

Fabulous recipes with mung bean sprouts include The Blue Healer (p. 112), Sweet Potato Toast (p. 123) and Cashew Caesar Salad (p. 170).

STORAGE

» Store mung bean sprouts wrapped in a paper towel in a sealed container in the refrigerator — they will last about a week but discard them if they turn brown.

» Always rinse them in water before serving.

How to sprout mung beans

Makes 1 batch, preparation time 5 minutes, takes 2–3 days to grow

Mung beans are one of the easiest beans to sprout and they are much fresher than the store-bought ones. Over the years I have found chlorinated tap water works best as it prevents the mung beans from going mouldy when they are left on the bench for a couple of days to sprout. You will need a seed sprouter or a glass container and netting or fine cheesecloth to cover.

- ⅓ cup dried mung beans
- ½ cup tap water (at room temperature)
- ½ cup boiling hot tap water

Sort the mung beans before use and remove the damaged ones that look darker or split (they won't sprout if they are split). After rinsing them with tap water, place them into a glass jar or container then pour ½ cup of tap water in, and then ½ cup of boiling hot water which will soften any hard beans (water that is too hot will instantly split some of the beans, so this ratio works best). Cover the jar with a piece of fine cloth or netting then secure with an elastic band. Set aside on the kitchen bench in low light, away from direct sunlight. Soak them overnight.

The next morning, drain the excess water and rinse the beans with tap water. You will need to rinse and drain the beans twice a day for about 2 days (they may sprout in as little as a day in very hot weather, and it may take 3–4 days in cold weather). You will know they are ready when the tails (roots) are about 1 cm (½ inch) long, and the little green shells have half fallen off. Refer to the photo on p. 32.

As soon as the beans have sprouted, drain any excess water, dry the sprouts and store them in the refrigerator, wrapped in a paper towel (or something to soak up the excess moisture) in an airtight container. Use them within 5 days for maximum freshness.

3. Beetroot (Beets)

Beets are the Red Cross of vegetables: ancient Romans and Greeks (such as Hippocrates) used them medicinally to treat skin problems, constipation and headaches, and the leaves were made into bindings for wounds. Red beets are a prominent liver and blood cleanser traditionally used to reduce jaundice of the skin, lower blood pressure and soothe digestive problems.[10]

Scientifically speaking, we now know that beets have potent anti-inflammatory, antioxidant and detoxification properties,[11] thanks to their unique betalain pigments, including betanin, which binds to toxins, enabling them to be eliminated via the urine. Beets contain manganese and folate and they are one of the rare foods that have a highly alkalizing effect in the body (boosting blood flow to your skin, which I find visibly brightens your eyes for an hour or so).

Consuming beets can sometimes make your urine or stools appear pink — it's normal and no cause for concern, but in some people pink urine (after consuming beets) can indicate high or low iron in the body (or malabsorption issues) so get your doctor to check your iron if this occurs.

RECIPES

Before artificial colourings became popular, beets were used to tint cake frosting, ice-creams, jellies and even wine. So let's go back to using beetroot to make healthy and delicious pink ice-creams, sorbets, smoothies and soups. Recipes include Banana Beet Nice Cream (p. 188), Pink Pear Sorbet (p. 196), Banana Beet Smoothie (p. 110), Beetroot Hummus (p. 145), Beet Cream (p. 163), Healthy Skin Juice (p. 116) and Beet Detox Soup (p. 149). You can also grate fresh beetroot into salads and wraps and use beetroot in alkalizing vegetable juices.

STORAGE

Remove the leaves and stalks before storing beetroots as this will increase the shelf life. Store the raw beets wrapped in a paper towel (to absorb excess moisture) in a sealed plastic bag or container in the refrigerator and they will last for weeks. You can peel them before use but it's not essential: just give them a good scrub and rinse them in water to remove any dirt.

4. Black beans (turtle beans, caviar criollo, frijoles negros)

Black beans are the superheroes of the bean world, thanks to their rich skin-protective anthocyanins, which make their skins appear black.[12] Black beans are a rich vegetarian source of protein, iron, vitamin B1 (thiamine), folate, magnesium, potassium, zinc and manganese, and they contain small amounts of omega-3, which is fabulous at decreasing inflammation in the body.

RECIPES

Add black beans to savoury meals such as Asparagus and Black Bean Soft Tacos (p. 155), Beet Detox Soup (p. 149) and Sweet Potato Boats (p. 180), or snack on Roasted Black Beans (p. 131).

STORAGE

If you are a busy cook like me you'll probably want to buy the organic canned varieties to save time. Cans are stored in the cupboard but once opened, rinse the beans, drain, and place them into a sealed container and refrigerate them for up to four days. Do not keep them in the can.

How to cook black beans from scratch

Sort the dried black beans and remove any stones or damaged ones. Using a large sealed container, soak them in plenty of water overnight (they will soak up a lot of liquid so don't be stingy).

The next day, drain and rinse the beans with fresh water. Tip: do not add salt yet as salt will toughen the beans during cooking. Bring a pot of water to the boil, then add the beans and simmer on low for about 45 minutes. Check them often. To gauge if they are cooked remove one and press it with the back of a fork — it should mash easily when it's ready.

Store them in a sealed container in the refrigerator and use within 4 days. Reheat them as needed.

5. Flaxseeds

Meaning *very useful* in Latin, flaxseeds were one of earliest crops harvested for making stunning linen cloth, paper and oil — and you can eat them too. Flaxseed is the richest source of plant-based omega-3 (even richer than chia seeds and hemp seeds) and it has potent anti-inflammatory, mood-boosting and skin hydrating effects. This little brown (or golden) seed is rich in vitamin B1 (thiamine), magnesium, manganese, copper, selenium and zinc and 23 per cent of the seed is gooey mucilage which can lower cholesterol and reduce diabetes risk and blood glucose levels.[13]

Flaxseeds, along with hemp seed oil, are my favourite dry skin remedies and they are both wonderful treatments for bumpy skin (keratosis pilaris) when consumed in your diet. If you are sensitive to flaxseeds (due to the content of salicylates or amines), use hemp seed oil instead (see p. 38).

Q: 'Are flaxseeds and linseeds the same?'

Yes, but 'flaxseeds' or 'flax' are terms used in relation to human consumption, and 'linseed' generally refers to industrial use (such as decking oil) or animal feed.[14]

RECIPES

Hydrate and soften your skin from the inside out by adding flaxseed oil to Papaya Flaxseed Drink (p. 116) and Banana Beet Smoothie (p. 110) or have ½–1 teaspoon of the oil daily (straight off the spoon) at breakfast — you can double the amount in winter if your skin gets super dry. Use whole flaxseeds to make delicious Carob and Flax Protein Balls (p. 136).

STORAGE

Flaxseed oil should be refrigerated at all times (except when in use) and used within 5 weeks after opening as the omega-3 oil spoils easily when exposed to air. Alternatively, buy flaxseed oil in capsules as the capsule coating protects the oil from oxidation.

Don't buy pre-ground flaxseeds as the omega-3 can go rancid once the seed has been ground and stored for long periods of time. To ensure it's fresh, grind your own flaxseeds with a seed/coffee grinder or a high-speed blender and store in a jar in the refrigerator. Make a week's worth at a time.

6. Hemp seed oil

Moisturize your skin from the inside out with hemp seed oil, which is a rich source of omega-6 (up to 62 per cent) and anti-inflammatory omega-3 fatty acids (up to 23 per cent). Hemp seed oil is rich in chlorophyll and vitamin E and has only trace amounts of salicylates, making it a good low salicylate option for people with eczema and chemical intolerance.[15] Do not cook with this oil as the omega-3 in hemp seed oil makes it unstable and easily damaged with heating.

While eczema is caused by various factors, a small study found that consuming hemp seed oil improved atopic dermatitis/eczema symptoms, while the olive oil placebo had no effect.[16]

RECIPES

Just ½ teaspoon of hemp seed oil (taken on a spoon) can give you softer skin in less than a week. But I prefer it in a smoothie to hide the flavour … recipes include The Blue Healer (p. 112), Carob Smoothie (p. 110) and Banana Beet Smoothie (p. 110).

Hemp protein powder is another ingredient I love — it's lean, green and great for strengthening your hair, nails and muscles when working out. It could contain salicylates and amines so don't overdo it if you have chemical intolerance or histamine intolerance (try the oil instead as it's purer). Use hemp protein powder to make Healing Hemp Smoothie (p. 109) and Hemp Protein Balls (p. 135).

STORAGE

Hemp seed oil should be refrigerated at all times (except when in use). Do not use it for cooking as heat damages it.

7. Leeks

Half a cup of leeks a day keeps the doctor away. Leeks are the mild mannered, low salicylate (and slightly posh) cousin of the humble onion, spring onions (shallots/scallions), chives and garlic. Leek won't make your eyes water but it does have wonderful health benefits to rival that of onions, including quercetin and other potent anti-inflammatory substances, especially when eaten raw or briefly water fried.

» Leeks are a rich source of kaempferol, which helps to protect your heart and blood vessels from damage, and science says leeks may lower your risk of heart disease, heart attacks and type 2 diabetes.[17]

» Leeks are a good source of allicin, which has the ability to reduce cholesterol and blood pressure and has antibacterial, antiviral and antifungal properties.

» Leeks are rich in prebiotic inulin fibre, which enhances calcium and magnesium absorption and feeds healthy bifidobacteria, allowing them to flourish in your microbiome.[18]

» Leeks supply vitamin K, omega-3, carotenes (which convert to vitamin A), calcium, folate, vitamin B6, iron, potassium and manganese, for healthy skin, eyes and blood.

The edible parts of leeks are the white and light green parts (discard or compost the darker green leafy top and roots). Leeks usually have dirt hidden in their layers, so unless you want gritty san choy bau, chop and thoroughly wash each leek layer before use.

RECIPES

Lovely leek recipes include Caramelized Leek Sauce, which makes everything taste great (p. 142), Oat and Leek Flatbread (p. 156), Sweet Potato Nourish Bowl (p. 169), San Choy Bau (p. 159), Cabbage Steaks with Beet Cream (p. 125) and Creamy Oat and Vegetable Soup (p. 177).

STORAGE

If you don't use leeks often, store them unwashed and untrimmed in the refrigerator. If you are a mad leek-aholic (enjoying ½ cup of leeks per day), pre-wash, chop and store them in sealed containers in the refrigerator for easy use.

8. Oats

Oats are the ancient healers of the grain world. Before the advent of scientific studies, ancient Egyptians, Romans and Greeks instinctively used oatmeal topically to treat skin inflammation. And you don't just smear porridge onto your face to get that healthy glow ... Oats, when consumed, have an important soluble fibre called beta-glucan, which lowers cholesterol and stabilizes blood glucose levels for a healthy heart.[19] Oat beta-glucan is wonderful for gut health too, working as a prebiotic to nourish and promote healthy bifidobacteria (in your microbiome) which can reduce the risk of colon cancer.[20]

So while grains such as wheat, corn and rice are getting a bad reputation, oats are still an ancient superfood that we can enjoy today.

Important tip: when using store-bought oat milk always shake the (closed) container to disperse the oat milk so it's creamy each time, otherwise it will seem watery. You will also need to stir homemade oat milk before each use.

TYPES OF OATS AVAILABLE

» Rolled oats (old fashioned oats) are where the groats have been steamed and rolled flat into flakes, then dried. These are my favourite as they are easy to cook and have a lower GI for healthy blood sugar balance.

» Oat bran contains most of the fibre from oat groats and it is the richest source of beta-glucan.

» Steel cut oats (Irish oats) have been cut into pieces — they are slower to cook as they have not been pre-steamed so they can be a little harder to digest.

» Oat groats are the whole kernel with the hard hulls removed — they are slower to cook as they have not been pre-steamed so they can be a little slower to digest.

» Quick/instant oats have been steamed, rolled and processed into small pieces so they cook faster and speed through your digestive system — this is not ideal as it means you will be hungry sooner than if you eat rolled oats, and they have a higher glycaemic index so they may cause blood sugar spikes (so favour the traditional rolled oats and simply soak them overnight for faster cooking).

» Oat flour: milling oats into oat flour improves the releasability of oat beta-glucan from 20 to 55 per cent.[21] Oat flour makes fabulous cookies and flatbreads, and you can buy oat flour online or make your own using rolled oats and a high powered blender (see the Oat Flour recipe, p. 42).

RECIPES

You can buy oat milk, rolled oats and oat flour, or make your own oat milk (see p. 42). Use rolled oats in recipes such as Overnight Oats (p. 119), Creamy Oat and Vegetable Soup (p. 177) and Papaya Sunrise Porridge (p. 120), or use oat flour to make Oat and Leek Flatbread (p. 156), Soft Tacos (p. 153) and Oat Bliss Balls (p. 135).

Skin care recipe: make your own blissful Oat and Zinc Bath Bombs to enjoy in a warm, relaxing bath (p. 75).

THE GLUTEN DEBATE

Oats contain avenin, a protein that has a similar structure to gluten. Most people who are sensitive to gluten will not adversely react to 'uncontaminated' oats, which are labelled as gluten-free in the United States. Oats in Australia and New Zealand are not permitted to have a gluten-free label (even uncontaminated oats don't make the grade in Australia due to the presence of avenin).

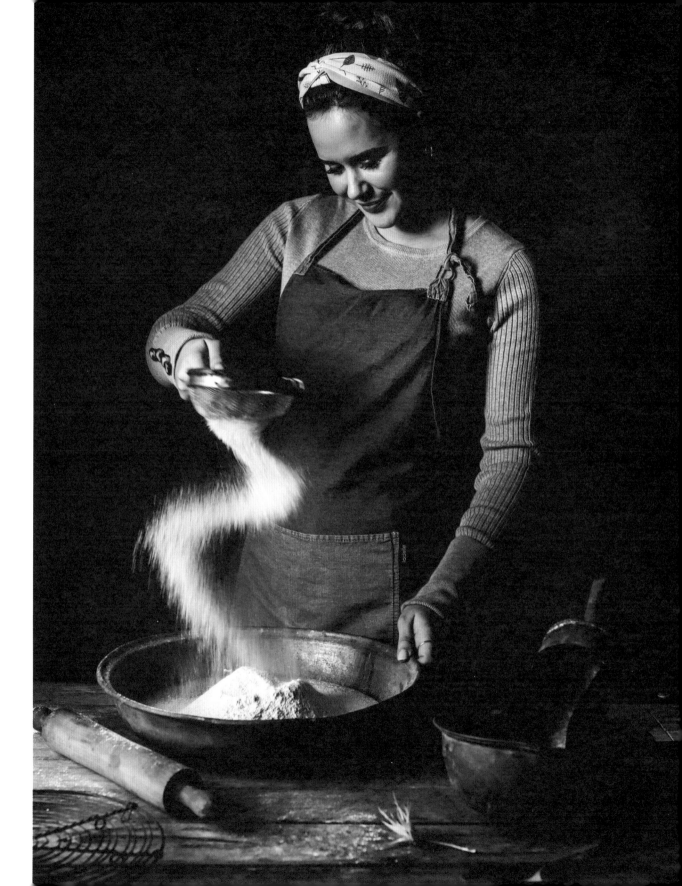

If you have coeliac disease or need to strictly avoid gluten, you might like to try gluten-free oats or simply avoid this ingredient. For the rest of us, you can rinse your rolled oats in water, strain and prepare them as usual. You can also opt for quinoa — it's a nutritious gluten-free seed that can be made into porridge or used like rice in savoury meals and salads. Recipes include Quinoa Nourish Bowl (p. 166), Quinoa Porridge (p. 120) and Quinoa and Chicken Salad with Beet Cream (p. 163).

Oat Flour

Makes 3 cups, preparation time 5 minutes

You will need a high-speed blender or a milling machine to make the oat flour.

- 3½ cups rolled oats

Depending on the machine you use, you will probably need to make this in batches, using 1 cup at a time. Mill the oats until they become a fine powder. Then use a fine mesh strainer to sieve the flour and, if needed, mill the lumps until fine. Store in an airtight container in the cupboard.

Creamy Oat Milk

Makes 5 cups, preparation time 15 minutes

A delicious, creamy plant-based milk (mylk) that is so good for you. Ideally use a high-speed blender such as a NutriBullet or Thermomix, but any blender will do as long as you strain the milk after blending. I usually make this without sweetener and add 2 scoops of calcium and magnesium powder to make it super nutritious, as calcium and magnesium are natural electrolytes which are essential for good health and strong bones. Oil is optional but it does help to reduce the viscosity of the milk so I recommend using it.

- ¾ cup rolled oats, rinsed and strained
- 4 cups filtered or spring water
- ½ teaspoon pure maple syrup
- pinch of quality sea salt
- 1 teaspoon pure sunflower oil or rice bran oil (or coconut oil if you are not sensitive to salicylates or amines)

You can make this in two batches if your blender is small or not high-speed. After you have rinsed and strained the oats, place all the ingredients into a blender and blend until smooth. If you are using a regular blender or a NutriBullet, stop blending and blend again a second and third time to make the milk smooth and creamy.

Then strain the milk using a nut milk bag, fine mesh strainer or cheesecloth. Add more water if you like a thinner consistency and more milk. Store in the refrigerator and use within 5 days. Stir the milk before each use.

9. Pears

Move over apples, the humble pear has won the award for the best gut-friendly fruit. The soluble fibre in pears 'sweeps' your bowels clean and helps to keep everything moving. The special fibre in pears also binds to bile acids, helping to remove toxins and chemicals from the body, which may be the reason it has a protective effect against some types of cancer, including stomach cancer.[22] In one study, the average daily flavonols intake was 14 mg — one pear provides about half of this amount by itself, thanks to the specific flavonol epicatechin, which has strong antioxidant, anti-diabetic and heart protective properties.[23]

Pears are a good source of vitamin C, potassium, copper, vitamin K and dietary fibre. They are gentle and soothing on the stomach, thanks to their low level of salicylates and amines, making them an eczema-friendly fruit and a wonderful first fruit for babies (after you have introduced mashed vegetables — do not give them fruit first!).

RECIPES

Eat your pears uncooked or make Overnight Oats (p. 119), Healthy Skin Juice (p. 116) or peel and freeze pears to create Pink Pear Sorbet (p. 196), Healing Hemp Smoothie (p. 109) and DAO Smoothie (p. 109).

STORAGE AND TIPS

» To test if a pear is ripe, press the very top of the fruit around the stem — if it feels slightly soft with pressure, it is ripe (even if the rest of the pear feels firm).
» Pears are generally bought unripe and perish quickly once ripe because they are low in salicylates, which acts as a preservative. So leave them on the bench to ripen and then refrigerate them as soon as they soften at the top.
» Rinse them before use.
» If you have eczema or are sensitive to salicylates (or following Menu 4), peel your pears before eating them as the salicylates are mostly concentrated in the skin. For the rest of us, enjoy the skin too.

10. Papaya

Papaya is the belly beauty queen of the fruit world. If you want a healthier gut, eat papaya as it's a natural digestive aid thanks to the digestive enzyme papain, which enhances protein digestion and kills parasites in your gut. If you've taken antibiotics, been ill, suffer from constipation or have leaky gut, eat a serving of papaya daily to promote bowel motility and recolonization of beneficial bacteria in the gastrointestinal tract.[24]

Papaya is a close cousin to the yellow pawpaw but it's sweeter and contains a red pigment called lycopene which, when eaten daily, increases your skin's resistance to sunburn (but still follow sensible sun protection guidelines when out in the sun for extended periods of time).

The seeds contain potent antimicrobial properties and they can be eaten to flush worms out of the bowel ('flush' being the operative word as they cause severe diarrhoea, so do not give papaya seeds to children or pregnant women).

One cup of papaya contains 100 per cent of your daily vitamin C needs, plus beta-carotene, folate, potassium and some vitamin B5 and magnesium for healthy skin. If you can't find papaya, buy pawpaw as they are very similar. Both varieties are easy to grow in the backyard in Australia and other warm or tropical climates.

RECIPES

Papaya is usually eaten ripe and raw with the skin and seeds removed. Try the dry skin remedy Papaya Flaxseed Drink (p. 116) and Papaya Sunrise Porridge (p. 120), Papaya Beauty Smoothie Bowl (p. 126), Oat Crepes (p. 195), Omega Skin Hydrator (p. 119) and Healthy Skin Juice (p. 116). Grated green papaya can be added to salads.

STORAGE

>   Always buy your fruits whole, not pre-cut, as fruit can develop bacteria when cut and left out of refrigeration on display at the grocery store.
>   Ripen papaya or pawpaw on the kitchen bench then store in a container in the refrigerator as they can perish quickly when ripe.

11. Chives

Chives are the classy cousin of the humble onion. Mild and pleasant tasting, chives are naturally anti-inflammatory and possess antimicrobial and antifungal properties. Chive extracts are used to relieve sore throats and sunburn[25] and chives are a good source of vitamin C, vitamin K, fibre, folate and carotenes which are converted into vitamin A, which is essential for wound healing and healthy skin.[26]

RECIPES

Recipes include Quinoa Nourish Bowl (p. 166), Beet Detox Soup (p. 149), Cashew Caesar Salad (p. 170) and Crispy Sweet Potato Gnocchi (p. 174).

GROW AND STORE

Chives are easy to grow and thrive in a vegie patch or a pot on a sunny balcony, and they repel insects in your garden. Chives also sprout pretty white flowers in autumn, and garlic chives provide a splash of colour with purple flowers. Chives don't last long once cut — that's another reason to grow them in your garden — but you can store them in a plastic container in the refrigerator for up to three days.

MORE WAYS TO USE CHIVES

Rinse in water and cut them into tiny pieces (I like using kitchen scissors but you could use a knife) and sprinkle them onto any savoury meal. They make a wonderful anti-inflammatory garnish for salads, fish, chicken, soups and oven-baked sweet potato. I love chives sprinkled onto Oat and Leek Flatbread (p. 156).

12. Spring onions (scallions, shallots, green onions)

What's the difference between a spring onion and a regular onion? Spring onions have no bulb — they are long and thin with green stems that are white at the roots. And you not only eat the white parts, you can enjoy the entire green stem too. The white part is best lightly fried (with water or a little oil) as it has some bite, but the green parts are mild and pleasant to eat raw or cooked — simply trim the root end and discard the roots, and finely slice the whole stem.

They are known by many names, depending on where you live: in Australia we call them shallots in New South Wales and spring onions in Queensland, they are spring onions in the United Kingdom and Singapore, and green onions or scallions in the United States. Refer to the photo on p. 28 if you are still confused!

» They are not just a popular soup garnish: spring onions contain a histamine-lowering, anti-inflammatory substance called quercetin which helps to protect against some types of cancer.[27]

» Like garlic and leeks, spring onions possess a potent antioxidant known as allicin which has antibacterial, antiviral and antifungal properties, all of which help to guard against Candida albicans in the digestive tract.

Spring onions contain vitamin C, folate, lutein and beta-carotene and mega-doses of vitamin K, which regulates calcium and assists with bone health and wound healing.

STORAGE
Spring onions will last up to ten days in the refrigerator if bought fresh and stored correctly. Cut the spring onions in half and store them in a sealed container (with a few paper towels to absorb excess moisture) in the refrigerator. Rinse them before use.

RECIPES
You can serve spring onions raw or lightly water fried in recipes such as San Choy Bau (p. 159), Creamy Oat and Vegetable Soup (p. 177), Sweet Potato Boats (p. 180), Lamb and Zucchini Pasta (p. 183) and Crispy Chicken (p. 184).

13. Sweet potato

Serve it up for breakfast, lunch and dinner: sweet potato would have to be the most versatile vegetable on the planet. Who knew sweet potato toast was a thing? Paleo people will do anything to get their toast fix, even whack sweet potato slices into the toaster — and it tastes great too, so I'm right on board with that. Sweet potato cakes, flatbread, vermicelli (from the Asian grocer), pizza base, soup, mash, fries, wedges, muffins and gnocchi — is there nothing this vegetable cannot transform into?

And it's a powerhouse of goodness too. One cup of baked sweet potato contains 770 per cent of an adult's recommended daily intake (RDI) of beta-carotene (which converts to vitamin A) and 65 per cent of our daily vitamin C intake. And it's a great source of vitamins B1 (thiamine), B2 (riboflavin), B5, B6, niacin, potassium, manganese, magnesium, choline and betaine, which helps to lower homocysteine in the blood. (High homocysteine is linked to increased heart disease risk, so anything that lowers homocysteine is brilliant.) Purple sweet potato can also improve liver and kidney function, which are the body's important filtration organs to remove toxins from the body.[28]

Regular orange sweet potato and purple sweet potato have an 'anti-obesity' effect, according to the research, so sweet potato is great for your waistline too. Researchers tested various levels of sweet potato in the diet and found that when 30 per cent of your diet consists of sweet potato, weight loss occurs and cholesterol levels plummet.[29] How do you increase sweet potato in your diet? Simply swap grains for sweet potato — for example, have a roasted sweet potato alongside dinner instead of rice or pasta. I've got lots of sweet potato recipe inspo for you.

RECIPES
Sweet Potato Flatbread (p. 150), Sweet Potato Boats (p. 180), Quinoa Nourish Bowl (p. 166), Sweet Potato Nourish Bowl (p. 169), Crispy Sweet Potato Gnocchi (p. 174) and Sweet Potato Toast (p. 123). You can also mash it or make sweet potato soup, instead of using pumpkin.

STORAGE
Wrap your sweet potatoes separately in brown paper bags and store them in a ceramic pot in the cupboard. Use them within two weeks, if the weather is hot. For sweet-potato-aholics like me, buy them fresh each week then pre-chop and store them in a container in the refrigerator for easy use.

14. Brussels sprouts
I used to hate Brussels sprouts (Mum used to nuke them in the microwave when I was growing up), but I learnt how to roast them and now they seriously taste amazing. And move over kale chips ... BS chips are even better.

You know they are good for you, but did you know they provide fantastic detoxifying and anti-inflammatory support?[30] Some of the ways in which Brussels sprouts provide this is through their rich supply of sulfur, glutathione, vitamin C and anti-inflammatory omega-3.

Brussels sprouts contain a special glucosinolate called indole-3-carbinol, which helps to prevent inflammation and cut cancer risk. Increasing your daily consumption of Brussels sprouts and other cruciferous vegetables (such as cabbage) can rapidly alter your gut bacteria so it produces more anti-cancer isothiocyanates.[31] Brussels sprouts also bind to bile acids, which has a cholesterol-lowering effect.[32] Half a cup of Brussels sprouts provides 130 per cent of your daily intake of vitamin K which is anti-inflammatory and plays a role in protecting you from age-related diseases including osteoporosis, heart disease and osteoarthritis.[33] And they have a cholesterol-lowering effect, especially when steamed.[34] It's the sprout that nourishes your whole body, so what's not to love?

RECIPES

Eat one Brussels sprout a day to keep the doctor away, in recipes such as Creamy Oat and Vegetable Soup (p. 177) and Green Detox Soup (p. 179). To learn how to make Brussels sprouts taste delicious, check out Maple Roasted Brussel Bites (p. 132).

STORAGE

Choose Brussels sprouts that are green and fairly smooth — avoid yellowing leaves that have perforations in them. Store them in the refrigerator in a plastic bag or sealed container, wrapped in a paper towel, for up to ten days. Rinse them before use.

15. Bananas

Pre-wrapped and ready to go, bananas are the 'fast food' of the fruit world. Packed with pectin fibre to soothe the digestive tract, bananas act as a prebiotic, nourishing the beneficial bifidobacteria in your microbiome which can reduce the risk of colon cancer.[35]

Green banana flour is another star ingredient and a wonderful flour replacement when making pancakes. Paleo people love it and it's vegan too. Green banana flour is a great source of dietary fibre and resistant starch, which has many health benefits including lowering cholesterol and improving insulin sensitivity which has potential weight loss benefits thanks to reduced fat storage.[36]

RECIPES

Make Banana Flour Pancakes (p. 195) or use regular bananas to make Banana Beet Smoothie (p. 110), Healing Hemp Smoothie (p. 109), Banana Bliss Overnight Oats (p. 120), Banana Popsicles (p. 191) and Banana Beet Nice Cream (p. 188). Or try Healthy Banana Bread — it's delicious hot or cold (p. 138).

STORAGE

Ripen bananas in a decorative bowl on your kitchen bench. Once they are ripe it's best to use them quickly or freeze them for later use. To freeze them, peel and discard the skin (or compost it), chop the banana into bite-sized pieces and store in a sealed plastic container or zip lock bags in the freezer, for up to three days. Use frozen banana to make delicious chilled smoothies and dairy-free nice creams (see below).

16. Carob

Hippies loved carob in the 1970s and you will too. I know cacao is trending right now (like carob was in the 1970s) but this is why I want you to get off that bandwagon …

Cacao is regular chocolate re-branded. It's loaded with adrenalin-spiking caffeine and headache-inducing histamines and it's a pimple waiting to happen (if you are prone to acne). And cacao can worsen eczema and dry skin. Carob, on the other hand, has been prized for its vast health properties for over 4000 years.[37] In the 1800s, carob was prescribed by pharmacists to soothe and protect the throat and alleviate diarrhoea (simply mix a tablespoon of carob powder with grated apple or pear).[38]

- » Carob is a naturally caffeine-free digestive aid that soothes and calms leaky gut and acid reflux.[39]
- » Carob binds to toxins in the bowel and inhibits the growth of harmful bacteria.[40]
- » Carob contains anti-cancer compounds and supplies calcium, potassium, magnesium, vitamin B2 (riboflavin), vitamin B6 and vitamin A for healthy skin.[41]

While regular chocolate can make you crave sugar (or more chocolate!), carob curbs hunger as it inhibits the hormone ghrelin, which makes you feel hungry.[42] According to research, ghrelin levels in saliva are significantly elevated in patients with atopic eczema (compared with eczema-free people).[43] This can make eczema sufferers feel hungry at bedtime or during the night, which promotes broken sleep.[44] Having a cup of Carob Tea (p. 115) before bed can help to promote satiety and better quality sleep at night. On the other hand, cacao could turn you into an insomniac if taken before bed, thanks to the caffeine. It's a no brainer — carob wins hands down.

RECIPES

Carob powder, carob protein powder, carob syrup and carob nibs are available from selected health food stores. Use raw or roasted carob powder (roasted gives a more chocolaty appearance) in recipes such as Carob Tea (p. 115), Carob Smoothie (p. 110), Banana Bliss Overnight Oats (p. 120), Carob Nutella (p. 141), Carob and Flax Protein Balls (p. 136) and make your own Easter eggs using the Carob Mylk Chocolate Bar recipe (p. 192).

STORAGE

Store carob powder in an airtight container in your pantry or cupboard.

17. Red cabbage

The superhero of the vegetable patch, red cabbage is one of the most important health foods grown on the planet. Red cabbage (which, quite frankly looks purple, not red), contains mighty cancer-fighting indoles and anthocyanins that help to lower inflammation in the body.[45] Anthocyanins not only create the pretty purple pigments that are absent in white or green cabbage, they also help to protect the skin against sun damage and reduce the risk of heart disease, diabetes, liver damage and some types of cancer.[46] One cup of red cabbage provides almost 50 per cent of your daily vitamin C requirements and it's a rich source of vitamin K, which is vital for strong, healthy bones. So it's worth switching to red cabbage to accompany your main meals. I have a cup of cooked red cabbage daily but any daily amount will do.

Cabbage belongs to the mighty brassica family alongside Brussels sprouts, kale, cauliflower and broccoli, but without the salicylates and amines that kale, cauliflower and broccoli supply, making cabbage a low chemical, friendly alternative. Traditionally cabbage was thought of as a medical treatment, prescribed for treating gout, diarrhoea and peptic ulcers.[47] And science has now proven the powers of cabbage in soothing peptic ulcers.[48] For centuries breastfeeding women have been applying green cabbage leaves to relieve engorgement, inflammation and breast pain. Today the humble cabbage leaf is a treatment that is still recommended by midwives, thanks to research that has proven it is effective at treating engorgement when the leaves are applied to the skin.[49]

RECIPES

It's easy to cook cabbage: just lightly steam or water fry the cabbage for about 2–3 minutes and serve it hot or try it raw in my favourite smoothie, The Blue Healer (p. 112). Cooked recipes include San Choy Bau (p. 159), Quinoa Nourish Bowl (p. 166), Healthy Fish Tacos (p. 187) and Sweet Potato Nourish Bowl (p. 169). Recipes with white cabbage include Cabbage Steaks with Beet Cream (p. 125).

STORAGE

Buy fresh whole cabbage or freshly cut cabbage that has not gone brown or mouldy where it was cut (this is important — mouldy cabbage can give you gas). Remove all of the darkest outer layers and wrap it in a long strip of paper towels, not plastic wrap (I find plastic wrap makes it go mouldy quicker). Store it in the refrigerator in the vegetable draw. If any discoloured patches appear cut them off and discard them — fresh is best. Use your cabbage within ten days.

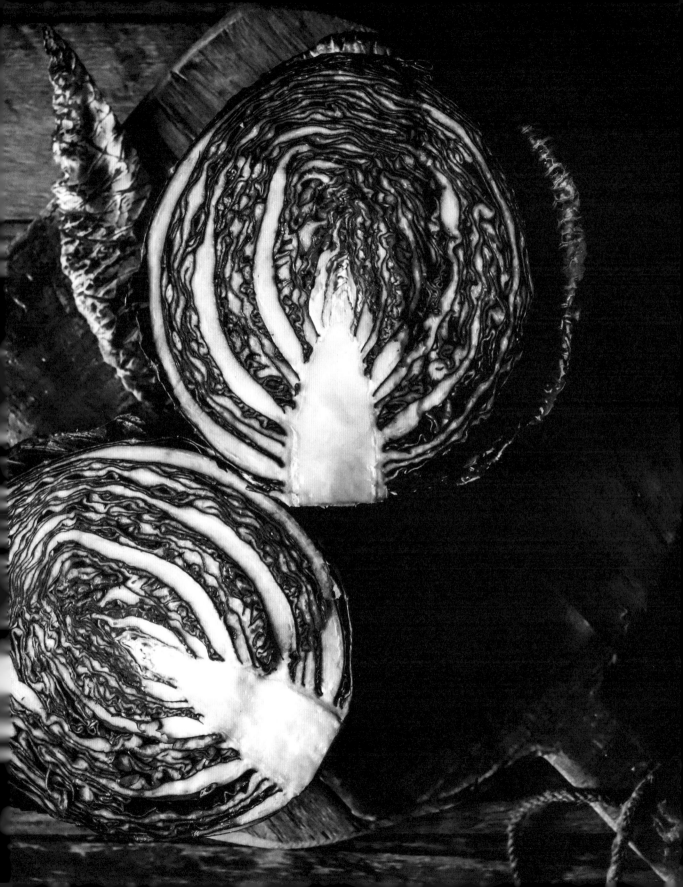

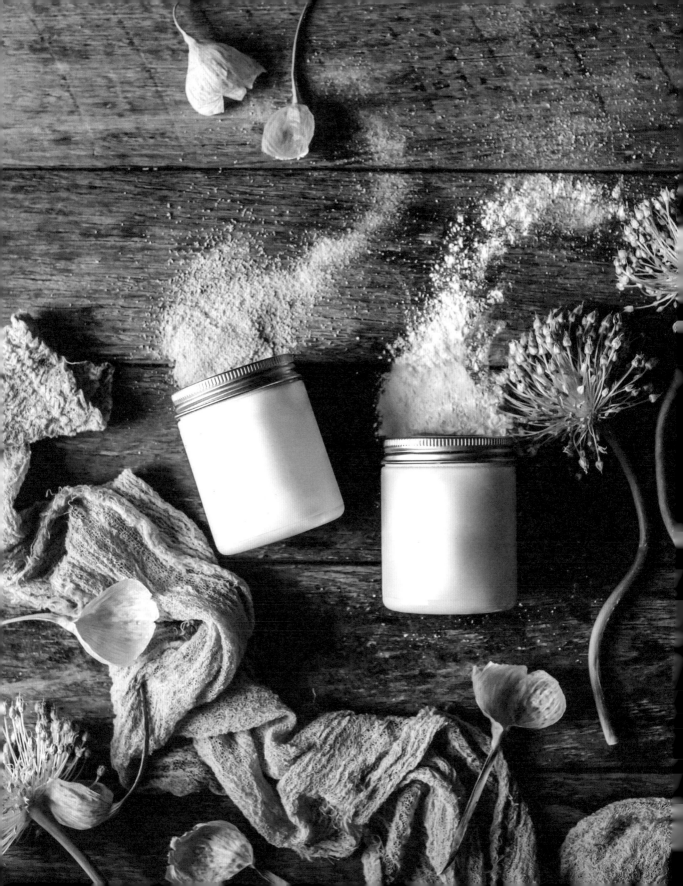

Chapter 4
Top 10 supplements for healthy skin

In this day of modern agricultural practices, where the land has no time to rest and replenish between each crop, healthy eating alone is often not enough to supply all the nutrients we need for healthy skin. Along with a healthy diet, I have seen supplements work miracles. Thanks to supplementation, I have witnessed skin disorder patients get their life back after years of social isolation and suffering.

Had I been well and energetic with clear skin for most of my life, I would have probably said, 'Supplements aren't necessary and let food be thy medicine'. Getting everything you need from healthy foods would be great, in theory, but when you have been on antibiotics or poorly fed or have crap genetics, good food is simply not enough.

While all nutrients are beneficial for good health, this book is about healthy skin so let's chat about the specific nutrients that are vital for getting that clear, healthy skin glow.

1. Vitamin C (ascorbic acid)

If ever there was a vitamin that proved without a doubt that your skin is made, modified and healed by nutrients, it's vitamin C. Scientists have demonstrated for more than a century that your skin literally falls apart if you don't consume enough vitamin C.[1] And vitamin C deficiency is not just an ancient sailor's disease, Americans today still suffer from scurvy according to the research — and it's usually linked to poor diet, poverty or fussy eating habits.[2]

But why I love this vitamin is its natural antihistamine properties, as it destroys the imidazole ring of the histamine molecule. For this reason it's imperative that allergy sufferers take vitamin C to avoid developing vitamin C deficiency. Some people with severe histamine intolerance (such as mast cell activation syndrome) may adversely react to regular vitamin C but they can try liposomal vitamin C as it is usually well tolerated (but check the excipients as it can contain soy). For the rest of us, ascorbic acid works well and you can also eat papaya, cabbage and Brussels sprouts which contain plenty of this skin-saving vitamin.

Vitamin C: dosages and food sources

Vitamin C (also known as)	Supplement dosages (milligrams per day)	Healthy Skin Kitchen food sources

Ascorbic acid
Calcium ascorbate
Magnesium ascorbate
  (may contain sulphites)
Sodium ascorbate
Liposomal vitamin C
	Children
	1–4 years: 35–50 mg
	5–12 years: 60–120 mg
	13–18 years: 60–120 mg
	
	Adults
	90–200 mg
		100 g (3½ oz) Brussels sprouts: 110 mg
		100 g (3½ oz) papaya: 60 mg*
		100 g (3½ oz) red cabbage: 57 mg
		100 g (3½ oz) white cabbage: 45 mg
		100 g (3½ oz) leek: 30 mg
		100 g (3½ oz) sweet potato: 25 mg^
		100 g (3½ oz) swede/rutabaga: 25 mg
		1 medium potato: 30 mg
		100 g (3½ oz) green beans: 20 mg
		1 banana: 15 mg*
		¼ cup mung bean sprouts: 3.5 mg
		3 spring onions/shallots/scallions:
		  15 mg
		10 g (⅓ oz) parsley: 10 mg^
		3 scoops Skin Friend AM: 120 mg

^Contains salicylates (not suitable if following Menu 4).
*Contains amines (not suitable if following Menu 4)

2. Vitamin B6 (pyridoxine)

I have a deep respect for vitamin B6: it's anti-allergy, liver and heart protective and a humble servant to aid magnesium absorption. Plus it's essential for a normal functioning immune system and good mental health as it's required by your body to make 'feel-good' chemicals, including serotonin. Deficiency signs include skin lesions, seborrheic dermatitis, cracks at the corners of the mouth, lethargy, sore tongue and dermatitis, which is a dry, scaly skin rash.[3]

» Pyridoxine is a natural antihistamine as it is needed to produce DAO, so it's a useful supplement for people with allergies and skin rashes.

» Vitamin B6 helps the liver detoxify chemicals by assisting the liver with deactivating and eliminating ingested salicylates, benzoic acids, food preservatives, monosodium glutamate (MSG), alcohol and heavy metals.

» Vitamin B6 is essential for normal fat metabolism and, as a result, a deficiency in vitamin B6 can raise cholesterol levels and cause fatty liver.[4]

A word against B vitamin megadosing

Supplementation of vitamin B6 is vital for people with skin problems but unfortunately most supplement manufacturers go overboard when it comes to B vitamins. They do this so you feel a buzz when taking the product, but it's not doing you good long-term. Less is more when it comes to healing your body. Below are some guidelines so you can get the best results from taking vitamin B6 for beautiful skin and a healthy body.

Vitamin B6: dosages and food sources

Vitamin B6 (also known as)	Supplement dosages (milligrams per day)	Healthy Skin Kitchen sources
Pyridoxine Pyridoxamine Pyridoxal Pyridoxine hydrochloride The active form that does not need converting in the body is called pyridoxal-5-phosphate (P-5-P): this form is needed for people with MTHFR gene defects	**Children** 1–4 years: 0.5–3 mg 5–12 years: 1.7–6 mg 13–18 years: 1.7–6 mg **Adults** 1.3–2 mg Therapeutic dose: 6–15 mg (do not exceed 20 mg per day in supplement form)	150 g (5 oz) grilled salmon: 1.2 mg* 1 medium potato: 0.7 mg 1 cup sweet potato: 0.6 mg^ 1 cup mashed potato: 0.5 mg 1 cup cooked lentils: 0.45 mg 150 g (5 oz) cooked beef: 0.44 mg 100 g (3½ oz) Brussels sprouts: 0.37 mg 1 skinless chicken thigh: 0.2 mg 1 medium banana: 0.35 mg* 1 fillet (127 g/4½ oz) flatfish/flounder: 0.3 mg 100 g (3½ oz) red cabbage: 0.2 mg 60 g (2½ oz) porridge/oats: 0.19 mg 30 g (1 oz) raw cashews: 0.16 mg (H) 1 cup black beans: 0.12 mg 3 scoops Skin Friend AM: 6 mg

^Contains salicylates (not suitable if following Menu 4).
*Contains amines (not suitable if following Menu 4).
H: contains histamine so not suitable if following Menu 4. People with severe histamine intolerance or MCAS may also adversely react to legumes, lentils and beans.

3. Biotin

Hello healthy skin, hair and nails. When I think of biotin, I think 'beauty nutrient' as it improves the thickness and hardness of brittle nails and helps to prevent hair loss and acne, when deficiency is present.[5] And did I mention skin rashes? Since the 1940s it has been well established that biotin deficiency can trigger the appearance of eczema, psoriasis, seborrheic dermatitis and oral dermatitis.[6] While not all cases of skin rashes are caused by biotin deficiency, this B-group vitamin is an essential part of any treatment program for skin inflammation because it supports skin health. Biotin from food sources is usually attached to protein and is poorly absorbed by the body, so biotin supplementation has shown to be a more effective remedy once deficiency signs have appeared.

» Biotin deficiency was found in 38 per cent of people with alopecia (non-hereditary hair loss).[7]

» Biotin stimulates epidermal cell differentiation and growth in the skin.[8]

» Avoid eating raw eggs as it can lead to biotin deficiency: the avidin present in raw egg whites attaches to biotin, which prevents its absorption.[9]

Take biotin with vitamin B6, magnesium and zinc to reduce skin inflammation, as together they aid the conversion of omega-6 and omega-3 fats into healthy, anti-inflammatory substances called prostaglandins (PGE1 and PGE3).

Biotin: dosages and food sources

Biotin (also known as)	Supplement dosages (micrograms per day)	Healthy Skin Kitchen sources
Vitamin B7 Vitamin H	**Children** 1–4 years: 8–30 mcg 5–12 years: 20–60 mcg 13–18 years: 30–60 mcg **Adults** 30–90 mcg **Therapeutic dose** 30–300 mcg per day in supplement form	150 g (5 oz) grilled salmon: 14 mcg* 60 g (2 ⅓ oz) oats: 12 mcg 1 cup sweet potato: 8.6 mcg^ 1 cup carrots: 6 mcg^ 1 medium banana: 3 mcg* 3 scoops Skin Friend AM: 60 mcg

^Contains salicylates (not suitable if following Menu 4).
*Contains amines (not suitable if following Menu 4).

4. Zinc

Zinc is one of those magic minerals that your skin absolutely needs for wound repair and skin health and maintenance. Zinc is essential for infant and childhood growth and development.[10] And during your teenage years, rapid growth spurts require lots of zinc and this growth period (teamed with a poor diet) can lead to zinc deficiency, which can result in acne. Acne occurs because the skin's oil gland activity is regulated by zinc — so *no zinc* equals oily skin and clogged pores that can become inflamed.

A healthy, zinc-rich diet is essential during your teen years and beyond. Unfortunately modern western diets that are dominated by packaged food, refined flour and sugar are linked with the increasing appearance of acne, according to epidemiological evidence, which shows that teenagers in traditional tribal cultures do not get acne.[11] But in Australia and the United States, even four-year-olds and mature adults are suffering from acne due to our poor diets. And this could explain why: zinc, magnesium, B vitamins and amino acids including glycine are required by the liver to *clear excess hormones* from your blood, so a deficiency in these helper nutrients can lead to acne, not the presence of hormones, which are a natural part of growing up. Let's look at the research:

» Early-stage zinc deficiency can appear as atopic dermatitis.[12]
» Skin lesions, dry and rough skin that looks like crazy paving, and delayed wound healing can occur during zinc deficiency.[13]
» Severe zinc deficiency can induce acne, blister-like dermatitis, nail changes, diarrhoea and hair loss.[14]
» Zinc gluconate supplementation has the ability to clear up inflammatory acne and treat hidradenitis suppurativa.[15]
» Zinc supplementation can be used to treat warts and leprosy.[16]
» Topical zinc creams can be used to treat warts and foul smelling sweat.[17]
» People with acne should avoid dairy products, chocolate and high GI foods that spike blood sugar levels (such as processed breakfast cereals, jasmine rice and sodas) as they can trigger breakouts.[18]

Zinc dosage — less is more

We as health practitioners love zinc — it's in right now. However, Scottish researchers found that 62 per cent of patients were prescribed *far too much zinc* by their health practitioner. The lack of understanding that zinc-induced copper deficiency can cause a range of serious health issues is far too common. Copper, while not a trendy mineral, is essential for collagen production and DAO enzyme production, which is vital to clear histamine from the body. Zinc can be your best beauty buy, but stick to the right therapeutic amount so the body remains in balance. See the following chart for correct zinc dosing and check the dosage before you purchase any supplement— even if it's prescribed to you.

Zinc: dosages and food sources

Zinc (also known as)	Supplement dosages (milligrams per day)	Healthy Skin Kitchen sources
Zinc gluconate (absorbed well) Zinc picolinate** Zinc oxide (used topically in skin care)	**Children** 1–4 years: 3–5 mg 5–12 years: 6–10 mg 13–18 years: 11–15 mg **Adults** 10–15 mg (no more than 15 mg per day in supplement form)	150 g (5 oz) beef: 7.7 mg 150 g (5 oz) lamb: 6.4 mg 100 g (3½ oz) dried beans: 3 mg 1 cup wholegrain oats: 6.2 mg 1 skinless chicken thigh: 1.3 mg 1 tbsp flaxseeds: 0.4 mg^* 28 g (1 oz) chia seeds: 1 mg^* 1 fillet (127 g/4½ oz) flathead/flounder: 0.8 mg 180 g cooked salmon: 0.8 mg^* 1 cup mashed potato: 0.6 mg 1 cup sweet potato: 0.6 mg^ 3 scoops Skin Friend AM: 10 mg zinc gluconate

^Contains salicylates (not suitable if following Menu 4).
*Contains amines (not suitable if following Menu 4).
**Note: I no longer recommend zinc picolinate. It is highly absorbable and as a result it can lead to zinc toxicity symptoms including vomiting, nausea, metallic taste in the mouth and copper deficiency.

5. Magnesium

Known as 'the great relaxer' magnesium is an essential mineral needed to keep more than 300 enzyme reactions working in your body.[19] It's one of the most important minerals you can take for good health and it could literally save your life. Why? Because you need magnesium to regulate your blood pressure, reduce the risk of blocked arteries and balance blood glucose, and it's essential for muscle contraction, energy production and bone development.[20] Magnesium deficiency can cause an irregular heartbeat (cardiac arrhythmia) and in some hospitals, magnesium is administered via drip to patients with atrial fibrillation.[21] Magnesium also helps to guard against asthma attacks,[22] especially when combined with vitamin B6 as it boosts the absorption of magnesium and helps to open the airways.

But let's talk skin health: magnesium could be your new bff because it helps you to manage stress and anxiety by lowering cortisol, the stress hormone that can lead to sleep issues and premature ageing. Magnesium also boosts beauty sleep — it regulates melatonin to help your sleep–wake cycle and it activates the parasympathetic nervous system to promote that chilled out feeling. If your body is low in magnesium, your cortisol levels stay elevated which can interfere with sleep.[23] Magnesium supplementation can be used therapeutically to decrease food chemical intolerances when combined with calcium carbonate, glycine and vitamin B6.

Magnesium: dosages and food sources

Magnesium (also known as)	Supplement dosages (milligrams per day)	Healthy Skin Kitchen sources
Best to worse sources: Magnesium glycinate (contains glycine to help improve sleep) Magnesium carbonate (highly alkaline) Magnesium orotate (very expensive for very little) Magnesium citrate (laxative effect, mostly citric acid) Magnesium oxide (very poorly absorbed, don't waste your money on this type)	**Children** (in divided doses) 1–4 years: 80 mg 5–12 years: 130–240 mg 13–18 years: 300–420 mg **Adults** 300–420 mg in divided doses	¼ cup raw cashews: 117 mg (H) 1 cup navy beans: 96 mg 1 cup boiled chickpeas (garbanzo beans): 79 mg 60 g (2½ oz) oats: 80 mg 1 cup cooked brown rice: 83 mg ⅓ cup barley: 81 mg 1 fillet (127 g/4½ oz) flathead/ flounder: 74 mg 1 cup cooked dried beans: 75 mg ½ cup black beans: 60 mg 1 baked potato: 57 mg 1 cup sweet potato: 54 mg^ fish (average serving): 26–50 mg 1 banana (1 cup): 41 mg* 1 tbsp flaxseeds: 40 mg^* 1 cup papaya: 14 mg* 1 cup Brussels sprouts: 31 mg red meat (average serving): 30 mg 1 cup mung bean sprouts: 22 mg 1 skinless chicken thigh: 16 mg 1 cup red cabbage: 14 mg ½ cup leeks: 7 mg 3 scoops Skin Friend PM: 300 mg 3 scoops Skin Friend AM: 60 mg

^Contains salicylates (not suitable if following Menu 4).
*Contains amines (not suitable if following Menu 4).
H: contains histamine so not suitable if following Menu 4. People with severe histamine intolerance or MCAS may also adversely react to legumes, lentils and beans.

6. Calcium

You could say that calcium is like Batman: ready to defend and protect your skin, bones and teeth. But even Batman needs a good wingman and it was Lucius Fox who made the Batmobile to transport him around Gotham City … without the Batmobile, how effective could Batman really be? Likewise, calcium needs magnesium (see p. 58). Magnesium transports calcium into your teeth and bones, where it needs to go, and without it calcium could be left floating around your arteries. So don't take calcium without magnesium — it's that important.

Together, calcium and magnesium calm the nervous system so you feel chilled and have a better night's sleep. But did you know they also play a starring role in the quest for beautiful skin?

» Calcium is needed for proper skin barrier function and damage to the skin barrier causes a decrease in calcium.[24] Defects in the skin barrier are seen in conditions such as eczema and severe dry skin.

» Calcium is needed to promote the 'acid mantle' (an acidic pH) on your outer skin layer, which is like the fortress that wards off microbes and infections on your skin. As you age, the acid mantle declines and calcium levels decrease.[25]

» Your skin must also respond to weather extremes, and in low humidity (dry weather) calcium helps to maintain the right amount of moisturising lipids by triggering their production when required. These lipids are water-resistant so they trap water in the skin so it does not dry out; so calcium is essential for people with dry skin.

» Low calcium levels in the epidermis layer of your skin hamper the natural exfoliating process so dead skin cells build up, leading to premature ageing and dry and dull skin.

Calcium to treat psoriasis

Calcium prevents skin cell build-up by increasing keratinocyte differentiation.[26] So calcium can be a wonderful treatment for psoriasis as it is a skin disorder, where the skin cells have poor keratinocyte differentiation and uncontrolled proliferation.[27] I used a combination of calcium and magnesium to successfully treat my psoriasis — only a low dose of calcium was needed and it worked quickly when combined with a healthy diet. If you are a smoker you need to stop that too, as smoking can cause psoriasis.

How much calcium for healthy skin?

The daily recommended intakes for calcium are very high and based on small, poorly designed short-term studies. In the United States and Australia, the recommended amount of calcium is 1000 mg daily, whereas in the United Kingdom 450–550 mg is considered an adequate intake for good health.[28] Considering how depleted most people are in magnesium, it's not advisable to take high doses of calcium. In fact, high-dose calcium supplementation will eventually cause magnesium deficiency, as calcium needs magnesium for its absorption. So for healthy skin, nails and bones, I recommend taking a calcium supplement *with* magnesium and get at least half of your daily calcium intake from food sources (see the table on p. 62). I prescribe calcium and magnesium in a 1:1 ratio (300 mg of each) so calcium is properly absorbed and there is no risk of magnesium deficiency — it's wonderful before bed as it promotes a good night's sleep especially when combined with glycine, which also improves sleep quality.[29]

Calcium: dosages and food sources

Calcium (also known as)	Supplement dosages (milligrams per day)	Healthy Skin Kitchen sources
Best to worse sources: Calcium carbonate (refined) Calcium carbonate (unrefined) Calcium citrate (mostly citric acid, good absorption) Plant calcium (from seaweed; avoid this type as it's rich in lead) **Note:** Calcium supplementation can interfere with drug absorption so take it more than 2 hours apart of medicines, and speak with your doctor before taking calcium if you are on medications. Do not take antacids containing aluminium while taking calcium.	**Children** 1–4 years: 300–700 mg 5–12 years: 300–700 mg 13–18 years: 300–700 mg from a combination of foods and supplements **Adults** 200–500 mg from foods and 300 mg from supplements Doses based on using a combination of calcium and magnesium for proper absorption of calcium.	1 cup fortified cashew milk: 300 mg (H) 1 cup fortified oat milk: 300 mg 1 cup fortified rice milk: 300 mg 28 g (1 oz) chia seeds: 177 mg*^ 1 cup cooked white beans: 161 mg 1 cup cooked navy beans: 123 mg 1 cup sweet potato: 76 mg^ 1 cup canned chickpeas (garbanzo beans): 77 mg 1 cup Brussels sprouts: 56 mg 1 cup leeks: 52 mg 1 cup cooked black beans: 46 mg 1 cup oats: 42 mg 1 cup red cabbage: 40 mg 1 cup papaya: 33 mg* 100g (3½ oz) beef, minced/ground: 28 mg 1 tbsp flaxseeds: 26 mg 1 fillet (127 g/4½ oz) flathead/flounder: 22 mg 1 cup cooked brown rice: 19 mg ¼ cup cashews: 10 mg 1 baked potato: 8 mg 1 medium banana: 6 mg* 1 skinless chicken thigh: 6.9 mg 1 cup oat milk (unfortified): 6 mg 3 scoops Skin Friend PM: 300 mg (refined calcium carbonate, magnesium glycinate, magnesium carbonate and glycine)

^Contains salicylates (not suitable if following Menu 4).
*Contains amines (not suitable if following Menu 4).
H: contains histamine so not suitable if following Menu 4. People with severe histamine intolerance or MCAS may also adversely react to legumes, lentils and beans.

7. Niacin (vitamin B3/nicotinamide)

Support mental health and wellbeing with niacin, which plays an important role in the wellness of your skin, digestive tract and brain. In fact, deficiency of this important vitamin can literally make you feel crazy with memory loss (dementia), diarrhoea and a skin rash known as dermatitis.[30] In the old days it was referred to as pellagra, which means 'rough skin', a disease that occurred in countries where corn or Indian millet (which are naturally devoid of niacin) dominated the diet.[31] Pellagra still occurs today in alcoholics, psychiatric patients, fussy eaters and people who eat poorly.[32]

Niacin deficiency signs include skin rashes, constipation, diarrhoea, confusion, red skin, headaches, digestive problems, mouth ulcers, memory problems, anxiety, depression and/or paranoia.[33] To diagnose pellagra, ask for a 24-hour urine test to check the level of N-methylnicotinamide. It can take six months to restore niacin levels once deficiency signs have occurred so if you have clear symptoms, nicotinamide supplementation is required as eating a niacin-rich diet won't be enough.

How much niacin is enough?

In the average person, 10–16 mg is more than enough. In fact, *less is best* when it comes to taking any B vitamin in supplement form as taking too much of one leads to deficiency in another B vitamin. And you need all of your B vitamins for a healthy body. Some naturopaths recommend doing a 'niacin flush' where you take high doses of niacin (up to 50 mg), which causes a whole-body hot flush as the blood vessels dilate. It's an uncomfortable experience that can cause a mighty migraine afterwards! But what flush devotees don't realise is it also triggers prostaglandin PGE2 production, which temporarily *increases inflammation* in the body.[34] So you want to take just the right amount of nicotinamide plus the entire range of B-group vitamins (from B1 to B12) so your whole body is in balance and inflammation is supressed. Most multivitamins and B-vitamin supplements contain far too much niacin and other B vitamins, which is why people with skin inflammation such as eczema can adversely react to these products. Use the following table to find out how much niacin/nicotinamide to take.

Niacin: dosages and food sources

Niacin (also known as)	Supplement dosages (milligrams per day)	Healthy Skin Kitchen sources
Nicotinamide (best source) Vitamin B3 (the old name)	**Children** 1–4 years: 6 mg 5–12 years: 6 mg 13–18 years: 10–16 mg **Adults** 10–16 mg (if you have eczema, take 10 mg in supplement form) For healthy individuals take 10–16 mg daily in supplement form	100 g (3½ oz) beef, ground/mince: 5.7 mg 100 g (3½ oz) cooked lamb chop: 5.4 mg 1 skinless chicken thigh: 3.4 mg 1 fillet (127 g/4½ oz) flathead/flounder: 2.8 mg 1 large baked potato: 2.1 mg 1 cup sweet potato: 2.7 mg^ 1 cup (81 g) oats: 0.9 mg 1 medium banana: 0.8 mg* 1 cup papaya: 0.5 mg* ½ cup Brussels sprouts: 0.5 mg ½ cup black beans: 0.5 mg 1 cup leek: 0.4 mg 28 g (1 oz) cashews: 0.3 mg (H) 1 cup canned chickpeas (garbanzo beans): 0.3 mg 3 scoops Skin Friend AM: 10 mg

^Contains salicylates (not suitable if following Menu 4).
*Contains amines (not suitable if following Menu 4).
H: contains histamine so not suitable if following Menu 4. People with severe histamine intolerance or MCAS may also adversely react to legumes, lentils and beans.

8. Omega-3

People with dry skin take note: you can quite literally hydrate your skin from the inside out with omega-3, a type of essential fatty acid that is, well, essential …

It's not just a beauty fad, omega-3 is absolutely essential for a healthy heart, skin health and mental wellbeing. Pretty skin is merely a bonus. And the research backs this up: scientists gave two groups of women flaxseed oil or borage oil for twelve weeks, and a third group received a placebo, which was olive oil. After six weeks of consuming only half a teaspoon of flaxseed oil, skin water loss decreased by 10 per cent. While the olive oil group had no change in skin hydration and skin health at twelve weeks, the flaxseed oil group had skin that was significantly more hydrated and smoother and the women had significantly less skin reddening after irritation.[35]

» Potent anti-inflammatory substances called EPA (eicosapentaenoic acid) and DHA (docosahexaenoic acid), which are omega-3 in its more potent form, help to calm skin inflammation, reduce skin sensitivity and enhance the immune system.[36]

» EPA and DHA are found in algae and seafood, especially salmon, trout and sardines.

» While omega-3 is essential, if you have acne you should get your omega-3 from fish and other omega-3 rich foods, and avoid oil supplements as your skin is already oily enough.

Omega-3: dosages and food sources

Omega-3 (also known as)	Supplement dosages (milligrams per day)	Healthy Skin Kitchen sources
Alpha-linolenic acid (ALA), also known as: linolenic acid **Note:** take vitamin B6, biotin, zinc and magnesium to aid the conversion of ALA into EPA, which is the active form of omega-3 that the body uses to make anti-inflammatory substances (PGE1)	**Children** 1–3 years: 500–800 mg 4–8 years: 800–1000 mg 9–13 years: 1000–1500 mg 14–18 years: 1200–1800 mg **Adults** 1300–2000 mg	100 g (3½ oz) cooked Atlantic salmon: 2260 mg^* 1 teaspoon (5 g) flaxseed oil: 2400 mg^* 1 tsp flaxseeds: 1140 mg^* 1 tsp chia seeds: 877 mg^* 1 tsp hemp seed oil: 875 mg 100 g (3½ oz) flathead/flounder: 563 mg 1 cup cabbage: 170 mg ½ cup Brussels sprouts: 135 mg 100 g (3½ oz) beef, ground/mince: 43 mg 100 g (3½ oz) cooked lamb chop: 175 mg 1 skinless chicken thigh: 99 mg 1 large baked potato: 15 mg 1 cup sweet potato: 7 mg* 1 cup (81 g) soaked oats: 81 mg 1 medium banana: 32 mg^ 1 cup papaya: 35 mg^ ½ cup black beans: 90 mg 1 cup leek: 88 mg 28 g (1 oz) cashews: 17 mg (H) 1 cup canned chickpeas (garbanzo beans): 45 mg

^Contains salicylates (not suitable if following Menu 4).
*Contains amines (not suitable if following Menu 4).
H: contains histamine so are not suitable if following Menu 4.

9. Molybdenum

Molybdenum is the great detoxifier. It is essential for liver detoxification as it activates the enzyme sulphite oxidase, which detoxifies sulphites (also known as sulfites) in the liver. When you don't have enough molybdenum to create this important enzyme, sulphite sensitivity reactions can occur such as alcohol intolerance, hives, wheezing, asthma, skin discolouration, eczema, dermatitis, swelling and diarrhoea (and in some cases, anaphylaxis).[37]

Molybdenum also helps the liver to safely metabolize drugs and toxins.[38] For example, if you have a Candida albicans infestation in your gut (from eating high-sugar foods), a toxin called acetaldehyde is produced during candida die-off. This toxin can cause fatigue, foggy brain function, joint pain and skin inflammation. However, taking molybdenum can reduce the adverse symptoms from candida die-off as it helps the liver to deactivate acetaldehyde.

Deficiency signs of molybdenum include intolerance reactions (to sulphites, alcohol, wine and vinegar), acne, allergies, asthma, rapid heart rate, multiple chemical intolerances and sensitivity to mould and yeast.

» People with gastrointestinal disorders such as Crohn's disease or gluten intolerance can end up with molybdenum deficiency.

» Take molybdenum along with vitamin B6, vitamin B5 and zinc to help your liver detoxify chemicals.

Molybdenum: dosages and food sources

Molybdenum (also known as)	Supplement dosages (micrograms per day)	Healthy Skin Kitchen sources
Molybdenum trioxide Molybdenum amino acid chelate If you do not consume legumes, you will need to take a molybdenum supplement	**Children** 1–4 years: 17–22 mcg 5–12 years: 22–45 mcg 13–18 years: 34–90 mcg **Adults** 45–100 mcg	½ cup lentils: 74 mcg ½ cup cooked dried peas: 73 mcg ½ cup lima beans: 70 mcg ½ cup black beans: 64 mcg ½ cup chickpeas (garbanzo beans): 61 mcg ¼ cup oats: 28 mcg 2 cups cos (romaine) lettuce: 5.6 mcg^ ⅓ cup barley: 26 mcg ½ cup chopped carrots: 3 mcg^ ½ cup chopped celery: 2.5 mcg 3 scoops Skin Friend AM: 80 mcg

^Contains salicylates (not suitable if following Menu 4).
If you have severe histamine intolerance or MCAS you might adversely react to legumes, lentils and beans.

10. Glutathione

If I were a cell (in the human body), this would be the love of my life. It's probably the closest thing to the fountain of youth that we'll ever find, as it helps to even out mottled skin pigmentation, reduces the risk of age-related diseases, reduces the appearance of age spots and calms skin inflammation (when combined with several other key nutrients).

Glutathione is a vital regulator of immune function.[39] It's often referred to as the body's master antioxidant as it's needed in most human cells to protect us from oxidative stress, which can damage our bodies like rust ages a car.

Glutathione is made by a healthy body from glycine, cysteine and glutamate. Your levels can fluctuate throughout the day and they are depleted by consuming tea, coffee, dairy products and most grains. Smoking, medical drugs and alcohol consumption also deplete your glutathione levels as glutathione is required to detoxify these substances.

I've seen long-term use of glutathione supplements remove uneven skin pigmentation and age spots — it's quite remarkable, but if you stop taking it the age spots quickly return. It's an expensive ingredient but what would you expect to pay for the fountain of youth?

Glutathione: dosage and food sources

Glutathione (best types)	Supplement dosage (milligrams per day)	GHS food sources (Jones 1992)
Reduced glutathione (it's simply called glutathione in Australia – ensure it's Setria)[40] Liposomal glutathione (beware of additives) Cofactors to make glutathione include selenium, vitamin E, vitamin C, riboflavin (B2), vitamin B12, vitamin B5, brassica vegetables (cabbage, Brussels sprouts)	**Children with eczema*** 150–200 mg **Adults** 500 mg In Australia, glutathione supplementation is not approved for use in healthy children as their glutathione levels should be good (but in unwell children it may be helpful)	100 g (3½ oz) veal cutlet: 26 mg 100 g (3½ oz) cooked asparagus: 22 mg^ 100 g (3½ oz) beef steak: 12 mg 100 g (3½ oz) baked winter squash: 11 mg^ 100 g (3½ oz) boiled white potatoes: 11 mg 100 g (3½ oz) chicken breast: 6.5 mg 100 g (3½ oz) raw carrots: 6 mg^ 100 g (3½ oz) Brussels sprouts: 4 mg 100 g (3½ oz) pears: 3.3 mg 100 g (3½ oz) banana: 3.3 mg* 100 g (3½ oz) cooked cabbage: 2 mg 100 g (3½ oz) baked sweet potato: 2 mg^ Have vegies raw or mildly steamed to preserve the glutathione

^Contains moderate salicylates (not suitable if following Menu 4).
*Contains amines (not suitable if following Menu 4).

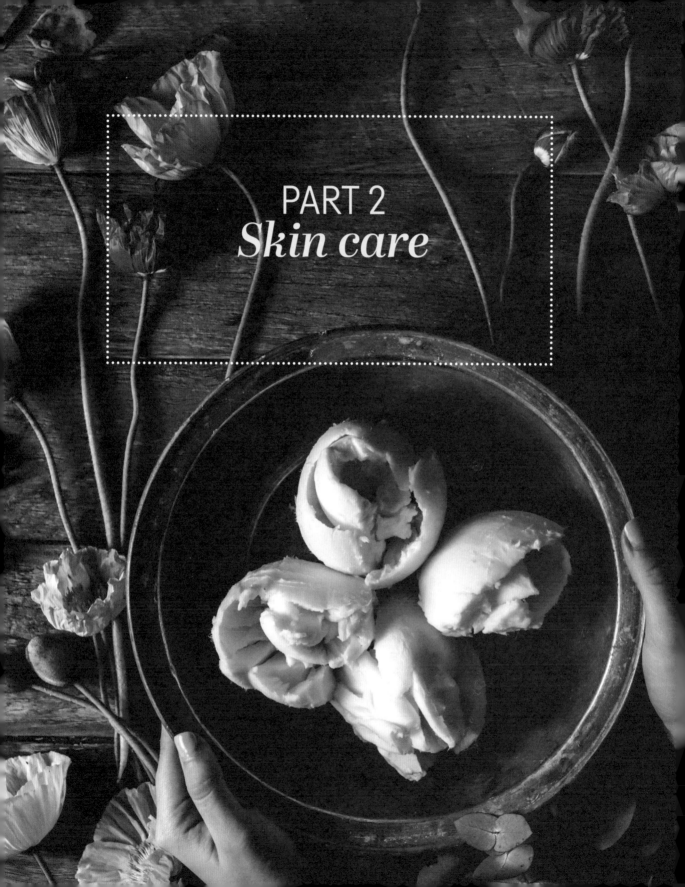

PART 2
Skin care

Chapter 5
Top 7 soothing skin care ingredients

I've had flaky, rash-prone skin from the age of ten and as an adult I could not find a single product to give me relief, especially during winter. For years I tested skin care products that were sent to me by companies for review (as I had a popular website called Health Before Beauty and had written *The Healthy Skin Diet*). Many of the products I tested had preservatives that I reacted to and herbal ingredients that were just too harsh for my sensitive skin. A few products my skin really loved but they just weren't hydrating enough for my dry, flaky skin.

To get the relief my skin needed I tested individual ingredients and products and found the ones that healed and soothed. After years of feedback, I know these ingredients work. Here are my top 7 soothing skin care ingredients for healthy skin — plus the skin types they are most suited for.

What is the difference between a cream and a balm?

Creams and regular moisturizers contain mostly water (and much fewer oils and goodies, so they are much cheaper to make) and they are ideal for people with normal or oily skin.

Balms and salves contain more hydrating oils and butters and less water, so they are perfect for dry skin types.

Ointments are usually water-free and may contain petroleum, lanolin and/or waxes and appear quite solid — they work as a barrier to lock in moisture but they can make your skin feel dryer afterwards, depending on the quality of the formulation.

A note on preservatives

Any product that contains water (which must be demineralized) or aloe vera must have added preservative to make it a safe product. I react to most preservatives (especially the natural preservatives, which can irritate sensitive skin), so natural is not always best. There are some great, gentle preservatives available but each person is different so patch testing a product before first use is the only way to know what is right for you. Some people prefer preservative-free ointments, balms and salves, which contain no water; but I found these are not hydrating enough for my skin, as a combination of water and oil works best to hydrate skin for long periods of time. If using these balms ensure you do not contaminate them with unclean fingers or water, as you will end up with bacteria in your product — this is especially important if you have broken skin such as eczema, which can easily get infected.

1. Evening primrose oil (*Oenothera biennis*)

Referred to as the 'King's cure all', evening primrose oil (EPO, for short) has long been used topically to heal the skin and enhance skin elasticity. It is rich in gamma-linoleic acid (GLA), which is anti-inflammatory and traditionally used to treat eczema and soothe joint pain and stiffness.

Ideal for: most skin types, normal skin to very dry skin, sensitive skin and skin rashes.

How to use: EPO is expensive and rather rich so it's best applied within a mix of water and oils in a *balm* for dry skin types, or a *cream* for people with normal skin.

2. Colloidal oat powder (*Avena sativa*)

Nature's soother, oats have been used topically for centuries to relieve itchy and irritated skin.[1] And today researchers have identified the active ingredients that make oats so special, including polyphenols called avenanthramides which are responsible for the anti-inflammatory and anti-itch properties.[2] Colloidal oat powder also contains cleansing saponins and beta-glucan, which forms a protective barrier to soothe and hydrate your skin.

Colloidal oat powder and oat oil are popular ingredients to soothe eczema, dermatitis and psoriasis, but anyone can use oat powder to cleanse their face and neck for glowing, soft skin.

Ideal for: all skin types, sensitive skin, acne and skin rashes.

How to use: Disperse oat bath powder into a bath or mix a teaspoon of oat powder with water to make a runny face paste to cleanse the skin (or remove light make-up by rubbing it in circular motions). Tip: Do not rub acne, apply oat paste and pat it on gently, leave it on for 1 to 3 minutes, adding more water to prevent it from drying out, and wash it off with water.

Home remedies: Make an oatmeal bath sock using ½ cup of rolled oats tied into a stocking/pantyhose foot or cheesecloth which you pop into a warm bath. Or make your own lush fizzy Oat and Zinc Bath Bombs using the recipe on p. 75.

3. Camellia seed oil (*Camellia oleifera*)

When trying a new skin care product or ingredient do a patch test first.

Camellia seed oil is prized for its skin restorative and hair nourishing properties and it's a treasured Japanese beauty secret which has been used for centuries by geishas. Cold pressed camellia seed oil is rich in vitamin A, vitamin E and squalene, which is a natural antioxidant that mimics your skin's natural oils.[3]

Ideal for: most skin types, normal skin to very dry skin, sensitive skin and skin rashes.

How to use: Camellia seed oil is expensive and works its magic within a mix of water and oils in a balm for dry skin types, or a cream for people with normal skin.

Home remedies: Pop a teaspoon or two of pure camellia seed oil into a warm bath and soak in it for 10–15 minutes (use a non-slip mat to avoid slipping and clean your bath afterwards). Or make your own hair treatment with camellia seed oil: massage it into your scalp and ends, cover your hair with a towel and wash it off after an hour, using a gentle shampoo and conditioner.

4. Refined shea butter (*Butyrospermum parkii*)

Shea butter is the superhero of the skin care world — it's not only super hydrating and anti-inflammatory, it contains antioxidants, fatty acids and vitamins which create skin softer than a baby's bottom.[4] It's extracted from the nut of shea trees and *refined* is better, as opposed to *un*refined shea butter. According to research, refined shea butter contains no IgE-binding proteins (the proteins associated with allergic reactions) which makes it allergy-friendly and unlikely to cause reactions in people with tree nut or peanut allergies.[5] I tested other nut butters including cocoa butter, and refined shea butter won hands down when it came to hydrating super dry and sensitive skin.

Ideal for: very dry, dry and normal skin types, sensitive skin and skin rashes (do not use on acne, oily T-zones or oily skin).

How to use: 100 per cent shea butter is too rich and hard to apply as it's solid — it works its magic when used in combination with gentle carrier oils (such as apricot oil and camellia seed oil) in a 'water in oil' formula, like a balm for dry skin or a cream or lotion for normal skin.

Home remedy: Pop a teaspoon or two of refined shea butter into a warm bath, mix until it melts, and soak in it for 10–15 minutes (use a non-slip mat to avoid slipping and clean your bath afterwards).

5. Sodium bicarbonate
(also called baking soda and bicarb soda)

Sodium bicarbonate is nature's exfoliator with antibacterial super powers.[6] For centuries, medicated baths have been prescribed to people with eczema and psoriasis, and bathing with sodium bicarbonate is a popular choice as it helps to reduce bacterial infections, skin itchiness and irritation.[7]

Ideal for: most skin types, acne and skin rashes (some people react to it when used 100 per cent on its own but are fine when used in combination with other ingredients).

How to use: Disperse ¼ cup into a bath or mix a teaspoon of bicarb with water to make a runny face paste to cleanse and exfoliate your skin. Moisturize your skin straight afterwards as it helps the cream to soak in nicely.

Home remedies: Make blissful Oat and Zinc Bath Bombs (recipe on p. 75). If you have eczema or psoriasis, combine baking soda in a bath with a tablespoon of oat powder and ¼ cup of apple cider vinegar for triple protection.

DIY Microdermabrasion recipe

Makes one treatment, preparation time 1 minute (plus 2–4 minutes application)

This is my favourite DIY exfoliation facial as it removes dead skin cells and leaves your skin feeling baby soft and smooth. It's ideal for most skin types, acne scars, enlarged pores, clogged pores, flaky skin and wrinkles and as a general beauty treatment you can do once a week. This treatment is not suitable for people who are sensitive to sodium bicarbonate or people with acne or rashes, as you should not rub inflamed skin (but you can pat the paste on, keep wet and gently rinse off after a minute).

Rinse your face and neck with water and semi-pat dry. Using your cupped hand or a small bowl, mix approximately 1 teaspoon of sodium bicarbonate (baking soda) with 1 teaspoon of water, then pat the paste onto your face and neck and gently rub your skin in circular motions for 2–4 minutes (avoiding the eye area), adding more water if necessary to keep it liquid. If it stings you can add more water to your skin or remove it sooner. Wash it off with water — tap water is naturally acidic and will help to balance your pH but if desired, make your own toner and use it to rinse your face and neck (see toner recipe, opposite). Then moisturize with a hydrating balm.

Toner recipe

Mix 1 teaspoon of apple cider vinegar into 1 cup of water and use it to rinse your face after exfoliation. You can place it into a spray bottle but do not spray your eyes — keep them shut!

6. Zinc oxide

Zinc oxide is nature's wound healer. It soothes the skin, has wound-healing properties and helps to protect against skin rashes such as nappy rash and eczema. It also has a potent antimicrobial effect when applied topically to the skin, guarding against Staphylococcus aureas (Staph), Escherichia coli (E. coli) and Candida albicans yeast infections.[8] It's also great on oily T-zones and is used in some sunscreen formulas as zinc oxide offers protection from sunburn and age spots, *when it is suspended correctly* in a well-made formulation.

Ideal for: acne (also refer to the acne treatment information on p. 80), oily skin, normal skin, dry skin, sensitive skin and skin rashes.

How to use: 5–21 per cent zinc oxide needs to be suspended in a mix of water and oils in a balm for dry skin, or a cream for people with normal skin. Do not use homemade zinc creams for sun protection as they need to be made correctly and tested for efficacy.

7. AHA and BHA

Want younger looking skin? Alpha hydroxy acids (such as glycolic acid, lactic acid, malic acid and citric acid) gently remove dead skin cells, making way for baby soft, younger skin. AHAs are used topically to treat acne, acne scars, clogged pores, wrinkles and age spots.

Beta hydroxy acid (salicylic acid) removes excess sebum and unclogs pores so your skin appears smoother and less oily. It's ideal for treating acne and clogged pores.

Ideal for: combination skin, acne, (also refer to the acne treatment information on p. 80) oily skin, wrinkles and ageing skin. Not suitable for sensitive skin.

How to use: Suspend within a mix of water and oils or in a serum. Use as a daily spot treatment or as a once-a-week facial.

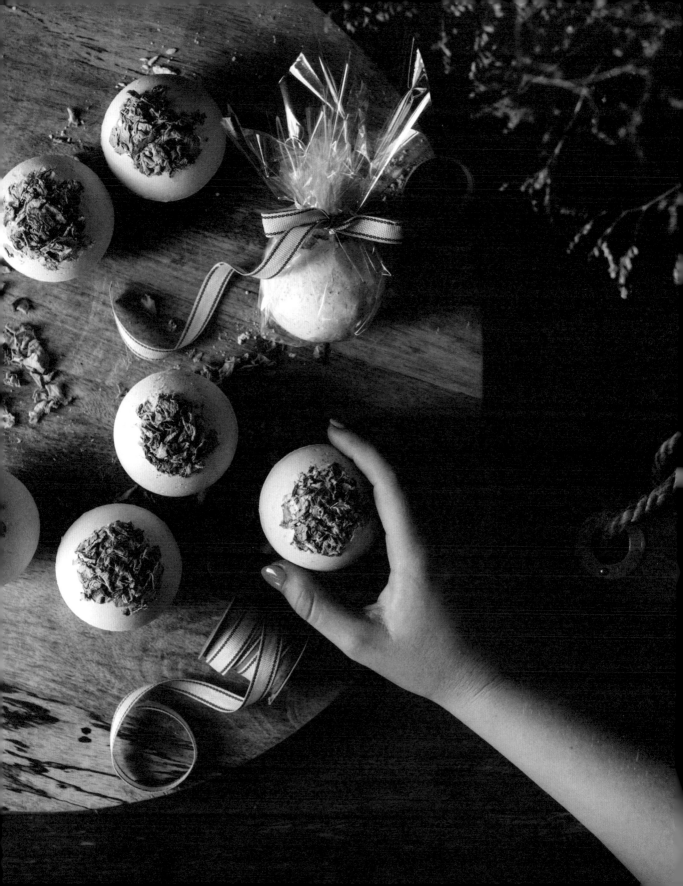

Oat and Zinc Bath Bombs

Makes 6 bath bombs, preparation time 1 hour plus overnight to set

There is nothing more relaxing than taking a warm bath with a fizzy bath bomb that is brimming with skin-softening ingredients. This bath bomb recipe contains sodium bicarbonate, zinc oxide, refined shea butter and citric acid, which is essential to make them fizz in the water. Citric acid is an acidic AHA with exfoliating properties that assist with cell turnover and the stimulation of new skin cell production.

You will need a spray bottle for the water, a teaspoon and at least three round stainless steel bath bomb moulds (stainless steel works best but you could use silicone or plastic moulds). Find an instructional video online at skinfriend.com (search 'bath bombs') or www.instagram.com/eczema.life and click on the bath bomb image.

- 40 g (1.4 oz) refined shea butter (about ¼ cup when well packed)
- 2 cups sodium bicarbonate (baking soda/bicarb soda)
- 1 cup citric acid
- 1¼ cups Skin Friend Oat and Zinc Bath Powder (or make Oat Flour, p. 42)
- water, in a spray bottle (or witch hazel)
- rose petals to decorate (optional)

Place two tea towels on a large tray (enough to fit 6 bath bombs) and set aside.

Using the double-boil method, place about 2 cm (1 in) of water in a small saucepan and cover with a sturdy glass bowl. Place the shea butter in the bowl and melt over a low heat until it becomes liquid. Remove from heat.

Meanwhile, mix the dry ingredients in a large bowl until lump-free. Then gradually mix in the melted shea butter, a drizzle at a time *to prevent over-fizzing your mixture*. The mixture should be crumbly and quite dry looking.

Now spray the water onto the dry mix, 2–3 sprays at a time, then mix. Be careful to not make the mixture too wet — it should still look pretty dry but hold together when squeezed into a ball in your hand (refer to the instructional video online if you are unsure). Spray 2 more sprays, mix, and squeeze a handful to check if it's ready.

Hold one mould cup (one half) and place approximately 1 tablespoon of dried rose petals into the bottom of the mould. Then add a small amount of mixture at a time into the mould and firmly press the mixture into the mould after each addition to ensure it is tightly packed. Repeat until the mould is full. Press tightly then continue to add mixture until it forms a pyramid/mound about 3 cm (1½ in) high.

Place this side down on the tea towel (to prevent tipping) and repeat the mixture-pressing process with the other side of the mould (do not add rose petals to this side). Once the second side is filled (tightly packed and mountain-shaped) bring the two sides together (over the bowl of mixture to catch spillage) and press them together, firmly turning and pressing as this will allow the excess mixture to fall back into the bowl. Continue to twist and push each side together until both moulds touch, creating a perfectly round ball. Continue to press them together to ensure the mixture holds together.

Now remove one half of the mould: holding the bottom half of the mould, use a spoon to gently tap the top half of the mould to encourage it to come off, tapping lightly around the top. Then gently using your hands, remove the top half of the mould.

Keep the bath bomb in the bottom half of the mould and place it onto the tray, using a tea towel to stop it from tipping over.

Then make the next bath bomb using the previous method. After half an hour you can take the bath bombs completely out of the moulds. To do this, cover the exposed part of the bath bomb with an empty half-mould, turn over the bath bomb, and use a spoon to lightly tap the other half to remove the top. Allow the other side of the bath bomb to dry for a half an hour. Once the bath bombs have dried on each side, place them onto the tray to dry overnight. If you live in a damp or humid climate, place your tray of bath bombs in the oven overnight — do not turn the oven on, it's just less humid in there (everyone can store them here, just in case).

Note that hot baths can dry out your skin so make the water warm (or lukewarm if you have eczema). Test it with your elbow before stepping in. Then pop a bath bomb into the bath and watch it fizz! Enjoy.

How to store your bath bombs: If you live in a humid climate the bath bombs will attract water and swell up over time so to store them, wrap them in clear cellophane and tie with a ribbon (as shown in the photo on p. 74) — this is a great gift idea! — or individually wrap them in plastic wrap and store them in a sealed container.

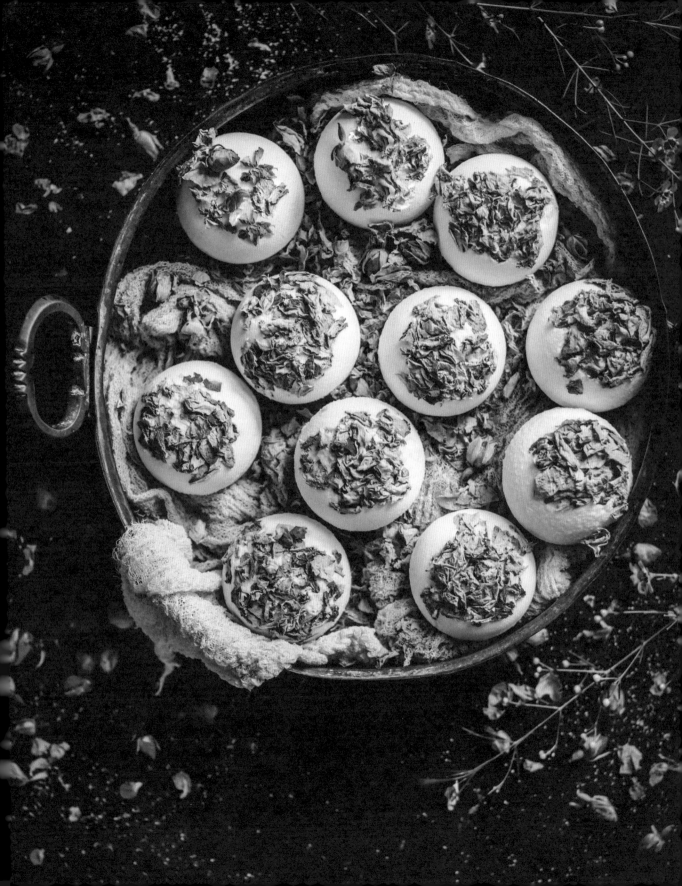

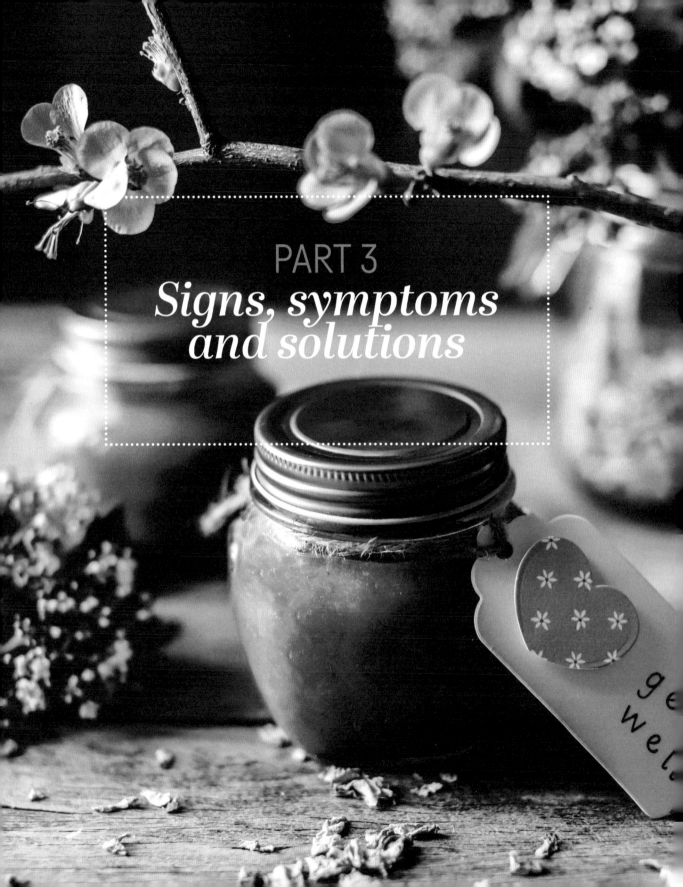

PART 3
Signs, symptoms and solutions

Your skin is a remarkable organ and your body tells you when something is amiss ... It speaks to you via pain cues, fatigue, feelings, hair and nail dysfunction and through the manifestation of skin disorders. Whether we listen or not is entirely up to us. You could suppress your body's cries for help by using a medicated cream (hey, we all need a quick fix occasionally) but it's also important to go deeper and investigate the underlying cause so your body can repair and renew and feel amazing. Part 3 shows you practical ways to treat and prevent skin disorders and associated health problems such as leaky gut — this is the section where you get to tailor your *Healthy Skin Kitchen* program to you. Enjoy.

Chapter 6
Signs, symptoms and solutions chart

Look up your personal skin/health complaint in the following chart to find the best foods to consume for healthy skin, hair and nails. Plus there is advice on supplements, nutrients and other therapies that have shown wonderful results.

The following advice is mostly tailored to teens and adults (especially the supplement dosages and recommendations) — and might be suitable for children when used in conjunction with a health practitioner's guidance (also refer to the supplement chapter for children's dosages).

Disorder	Causes/triggers; foods to avoid	Treatments and diet
Acne/pimples Inflammatory skin disorder where the sebaceous glands produce too much oil and the hair follicles become clogged with oil and dead skin cells	**Triggers**: modern western diets (rich in sugar and refined grains), dairy products, farmed milk (rich in steroid hormones), stress, nutritional deficiencies including zinc, B vitamins and magnesium **Foods to avoid**: junk food, sweets, dairy products, chocolate, almonds and most nuts, cooking oils (with the exception of olive oil), deli meats, bacon, high GI foods (pumpkin, most breakfast cereals), jasmine rice, flaxseed oil, hemp seed oil, chia seeds, dates and dried fruits	**Food:** fresh vegetables, lean meats, extra virgin olive oil, fish, legumes, oats and papaya. Refer to Menu 1 (p. 97); sip 3L (6.3 pt) of water daily **Supplements:** 10–15 mg zinc, nicotinamide (B3), biotin, pantothenic acid (B5), pyridoxine (B6) and magnesium (Skin Friend AM) **Skin care:** Synergie Skin (ReVeal, Blem-X); Skin Friend Oat and Zinc Bath Powder
Alopecia (hair loss) T-cell mediated autoimmune disorder of the hair follicles (not hereditary baldness in men)	**Triggers:** autoimmune disorders, trauma, stress, anxiety, mast cell activation syndrome (p. 87), red skin syndrome (TSW), nutritional deficiencies including biotin, iron, zinc, amino acids (protein) and essential fatty acids such as omega-3 and omega-6	**Food:** protein powder to stop the hair loss (pea, rice or hemp protein powder), refer to menus 2 and 3 (pp. 98–99) **Supplements:** 1 tsp flaxseed oil or hemp seed oil daily; biotin, zinc, vitamin B6, magnesium and 500 mg glutathione **Other:** manage stress with daily 20-minute meditation and 10 minutes of deep breathing (refer to vagal tone, p. 18). Camellia seed oil to help regrow hair and nourish the scalp with essential fatty acids (apply it 3 nights per week and rinse in the morning)

Candidiasis

Candida albicans overgrowth/ infestation

Yeast infection

Thrush

Oral thrush (white patches on the tongue)

Triggers: excess antibiotic use (2 courses in a row), sugar/ sweetener consumption (yeast needs sugar to survive), too much fruit in the diet, stress (for example, anxiety when beginning a new intimate relationship), unhealthy microbiome caused by excess consumption of sweet foods, dried fruits and processed grains

Advice: Avoid baths and swimming if possible, avoid wearing wet swimwear for extended periods of time

Usually kept under control by a healthy microbiome (p. 11), a short fast can help (see p. 12)

Food: avoid eating sweet foods until symptoms subside for at least a month; eat vegetables, meats and legumes (limit grains to oats or red quinoa); sip 3L (6.3 pt) of water daily.

Oral supplements: molybdenum, magnesium and biotin (Skin Friend AM)

Other: antifungal medications if necessary (fluconazole/nystatin tablets or oral liquid); avoid antibiotics unless absolutely necessary; when starting a new relationship, wait until you feel trust and are deeply connected to a person before having sex for the first time

Cellulite

Dimpling of the skin, thighs, bottom and abdomen

If you are a woman, it takes ongoing commitment and effort to prevent cellulite with daily exercise and a strict diet. You can get rid of cellulite but the sacrifices you need to make might be too much for some people. If you enjoy fitness, you'll find this rewarding. Treat cellulite from a place of self-love, not self-loathing. You'll succeed if self-love is your motivation.

Triggers: modern western diets, dairy products, sugar and starchy foods, sedentary lifestyle, calcium deficiency, salt excess, excess histamines in the diet, excess weight

Foods to avoid: dairy products, sweetened foods (anything addictive), wheat, most grains (except oats), fast food, junk food, alcohol, high GI foods such as rice, processed breakfast cereal and pumpkin

Food: Papaya Flaxseed Drink (p. 116), vegetables, lean meats and fresh fish (refer to Menu 2, p. 98)

Supplements: hemp protein powder (Healing Hemp Smoothie p. 109), calcium and magnesium (Skin Friend PM), zinc, silica, vitamin C (Skin Friend AM)

Other: 40–60 minutes daily exercise (e.g. yoga, Pilates, barre, HIIT, soft sand walking/jogging, lifting weights, booty workouts)

Cellulitis

Infected skin rash (such as eczema) that is painful, inflamed, swollen and red or purple in colour; smelly eczema is a sign of infection (may smell like rotting meat)

Triggers: scratching itchy skin, broken skin such as eczema becomes infected with bacteria

Infections can be dangerous if left untreated so see your doctor as antibiotics are essential to treat cellulitis

Skin care as a preventative: zinc oxide is antibacterial

Chronic inflammatory response syndrome (CIRS)

Mould sickness and exposure to biotoxins: symptoms include skin sensitivity, skin rashes, pins and needles/tingling skin, poor concentration, asthma, abdominal pains, cough, numbness, diarrhoea, poor memory, shortness of breath, congested sinuses, metallic taste in mouth, watery eyes, weakness, body aches, headaches, sensitivity to light, poor learning, night sweats, mood swings, pain, bloodshot eyes, morning stiffness, joint pain, muscle cramps, chronic fatigue, dizziness, static shocks, extreme thirst, cough, confusion, trouble regulating body temperature, frequent urination

Triggers: 25% of people are sensitive to exposure to mould and other biotoxins; water damaged buildings, contaminated reef fish, tick bites (Lyme disease) and recluse spider bites

Identify and remove triggers (remove mould from home and throw away mouldy clothes and books; clean furniture and enlist specialist advice; clean air-conditioners, remove old carpet if necessary), buy an air purifier with a HEPA filter to clean air

Check for MCAS (p. 87) as it can occur with CIRS

For diagnosis, begin with online VCS screening test (survivingmold.com);
Supplements: 500 mg glutathione daily (liposomal or reduced glutathione, no flavouring);
Food: ½ tsp hemp seed oil or flaxseed oil; low histamine diet; 3L (6.3 pt) water daily; begin with Menu 4 (p. 100), and progress to Menu 3 (p. 99)
Other: avoid stress; improve vagal tone (p. 18); speak to a practitioner trained by Dr Shoemaker (survivingmold.com) as there are medications that can be prescribed, such as cholestyramine, which binds to mould and removes it via your bile; DNRS training (see 'Helpful resources', p. 198) if necessary

Dandruff

Flaky scalp associated with psoriasis, seborrheic dermatitis, eczema and fungal infections

Triggers: nutritional deficiencies including omega-3 essential fatty acids, zinc, biotin and other B vitamins and selenium; stress, harsh shampoos (sodium lauryl sulfate/SLS and sodium laureth sulfate/SLES), chemical sensitivity

Supplements: biotin, zinc, vitamin B6 (Skin Friend AM); omega-3 (1 tsp flaxseed oil or hemp seed oil daily)
Hair care: fill a spray bottle with water, ¼ cup apple cider vinegar and ½ tsp pure vitamin E oil. Shake and spray onto your scalp before bed. Wash your hair in the morning. Use daily or as needed. Use gentle shampoo and conditioners (avoid dyes, SLS and SLES)

Dermatitis (all types)
Skin rash: types include atopic dermatitis/eczema, seborrheic dermatitis, contact dermatitis, neurodermatitis (lichen simplex chronicus), perioral dermatitis

(also see Eczema p. 84)

Triggers: *Contact dermatitis* triggers include chemicals, cheap jewellery, perfume, hair dye, poison ivy, latex etc.

Seborrheic dermatitis and dermatitis triggers include deficiency in biotin, zinc, niacin, vitamin B12 and/or vitamin B6[1] (deficiency caused by poor diet, some medical drugs, alcohol consumption, yeast infection and illness)

Neurodermatitis is caused by scratching and B vitamin deficiencies (see above)

Perioral dermatitis is caused by nutritional deficiencies (see above) food sensitivities, nasal sprays and corticosteroid inhalers

Food: see Menu 3, p. 99
Supplements: vitamin B12, biotin, niacin, zinc and vitamin B6 (Skin Friend AM); 1 tsp flaxseed oil or hemp seed oil (omega-3, see p. 64); glutathione and magnesium, low dose B vitamins, zinc, molybdenum (Skin Friend AM)
For improving sleep: calcium and magnesium (Skin Friend PM)
Clothing: soft bamboo and/or 100% cotton clothing and bedding
Skin care: Skin Friend 24-Hour Rescue Balm, Skin Friend Oat and Zinc Bath Powder
Important: if your rash smells bad your skin could be infected (see Cellulitis p. 81)

Dry skin (very dry and flaking skin)
filaggrin gene defects
Flaky and rough skin
Cracked skin

Filaggrin gene defect signs include dry skin, hyper-lined creases in palms of hands, rashes on hands, eczema, thickened skin on backs of hands, wrinkly hands (in young people), chapped hands (worse in winter)

Triggers: genetic defect/loss of function in the filaggrin genes (increases skin pH and decreases skin hydration), stress, poor diet, omega-3 deficiency, omega-6 imbalance, calcium deficiency, dehydration

Food: chia seeds, flaxseeds; menus 2 or 3 (see p. 98–99); See The Blue Healer (p. 112) or Papaya Flaxseed Drink (p. 116)
Supplements: ½–1 tsp hemp seed oil or flaxseed oil, and calcium; drink 3L (6.3 pt) of water daily
Skin care: Skin Friend 24-Hour Rescue Balm to help restore skin barrier function

Eczema (all types)

Deeply itchy skin rash, which can weep, crust and flake
Types include atopic eczema (atopic dermatitis), asteatotic eczema, discoid eczema, gravitational eczema (varicose eczema; stasis eczema), pompholyx eczema (dyshidrotic eczema)

Differential diagnosis: severe/chronic eczema can be caused by an autoimmune response such as MCAS (p. 87) or CIRS (p. 82) so read about them to check if they apply to you

When you are itchy, check your last thoughts: were you stressed, anxious, negative, judgmental or unkind to yourself? Whenever you itch, practice *gratitude* by listing everything you are grateful for until you feel warm and fuzzy inside. Keep going until the itch goes away – gratitude releases anti-inflammatory, pain-numbing chemicals in the body that can stop the itch

Triggers: genetic predisposition, stress, anxiety, food intolerances, allergies, Candida albicans infection, gut dysbiosis, self-criticism, salicylate intolerance, stress triggered by violence on TV/games as the body cannot distinguish between real and imagined, histamine intolerance, filaggrin gene defects (p. 83)
(If eczema *weeps/oozes* it's usually triggered by something you ate that day ... for me this was legumes)
Foods to avoid: dairy products, chocolate, alcohol, wheat, most grains (except oats, rice, tapioca, and quinoa), fast food, junk food, processed breakfast cereal, yoghurt, dried fruits, avocado, coconut, mushrooms, corn, dark leafy green vegies (if salicylate intolerant), deli meats, bacon, ham, sausages, sauces
Advice: learn to relax and meditate to calm your nervous system

Food: drink 3L (6.3 pt) of water daily (healing can only occur when you are hydrated), eat a diet low in salicylates and histamines to see if this helps, begin on Menu 4 (p. 100) and progress to Menu 3 (p. 99)
Supplements: ½–1 tsp of flaxseed oil or hemp seed oil (see omega-3 information, p. 64); glutathione, biotin, magnesium, low dose B vitamins, zinc, molybdenum (Skin Friend AM); to improve sleep: calcium and magnesium (Skin Friend PM)
Clothing: soft bamboo and/or 100% cotton clothing and bedding (400 thread count sheets, not higher); read information on vagal tone (p. 18) to calm down your nervous system
Skin care: Skin Friend 24-Hour Rescue Balm, Skin Friend Oat and Zinc Bath Powder
Other: if your eczema smells bad your skin could be infected so read 'Cellulitis', p. 81, and have your doctor check for infection

Hidradenitis suppurativa

Small red, painful lumps under the skin that can break open and form tunnels into the skin, may look like boils

Triggers: smoking, obesity, poor diet, sensitivity to dairy products (milk, yoghurt, cheese, butter), sugary foods, refined grains (pasta, wheat flour, pizza, doughnuts, cakes, biscuits), potato chips, fries, alcohol, nightshades (tomato, eggplant/aubergine, white potato, capsicum/peppers, goji berries)
Advice: quit smoking, avoid alcohol, lose weight (if needed), eat healthy food, avoid sugar and dairy

Food: Papaya Flaxseed Drink (p. 116), Healing Hemp Smoothie (p. 109), The Blue Healer (p. 112); see Menu 1 (p. 97) and Menu 3 (p. 99); drink 3L (6.3 pt) of water daily
Supplements: Skin Friend AM
Skin care: soak in a bath with Skin Friend Oat and Zinc Bath Powder and ¼ cup apple cider vinegar, twice a week
Clothing: if needed, wear loose 100% cotton or bamboo clothing and bedding (400 thread count sheets, no higher as they can trap too much heat)

Histamine/amine intolerance
Histamine toxicity:
associated with MCAS
(p. 87), rosacea, eczema, hives,
itchy skin, swelling, low blood
pressure, rapid heartbeat, chest
pains, headaches, fatigue,
digestive tract upsets, reflux,
rhinitis, nutritional deficiencies

Triggers: stress, nutritional
deficiencies including vitamin C,
copper, vitamin B6, MCAS
(p. 87), bacteria in the microbiome
producing high histamine; excess
consumption of high histamine
foods (fermented foods, ungutted/
bad fish, shellfish, cheese, leftover
meats, vinegar, yoghurt, soy sauce,
deli meats and alcohol) plus DAO
deficiency

Food: Menu 4 (p. 100) is a low histamine
diet program
Supplements: take DAO nutrients vitamin
C, vitamin B6 (Skin Friend AM), copper
(if deficient), quercetin (if tolerated); drink
the DAO Smoothie (p. 109); avoid alcohol;
test 1 course of histamine-lowering
probiotic (caution, probiotics may worsen
symptoms and are not suitable for
everyone)
Refer to MCAS treatments on p. 87 for
more advice

Hives (urticaria)
Red, raised welts that can be
itchy, they can present as tiny
dots, the size of a mosquito bite,
up to very large round welts the
size of a small plate

Triggers: stress, anxiety, worry,
food intolerances, allergies, MCAS
(p. 87), CIRS (p. 82), cold weather,
weather extremes, cold water,
electromagnetic sensitivity
Foods to avoid: high histamine
foods, see 'Helpful resources', p. 198
and check for salicylate intolerance
or other food intolerances

Food: The Blue Healer (p. 112), low
salicylate and low histamine foods
(see Menu 4, p. 100)
sip 3L (6.3 pt) of water daily
Supplements: ½–1 tsp of flaxseed oil
or hemp seed oil (omega-3, see p. 64);
glutathione, biotin, magnesium, zinc,
(Skin Friend AM); for improving sleep:
calcium and magnesium (Skin Friend
PM)
Clothing: soft bamboo and/or 100%
cotton clothing and bedding
Skin care: Skin Friend 24-Hour Rescue
Balm; Skin Friend Oat and Zinc Bath
Powder
Check vagal tone (p. 18) and microbiome
(p. 11)

Keratosis pilaris
Sometimes referred to as
chicken skin, as a build-up of
keratin in the skin makes it
appear like red goose bumps
that become inflamed and
irritated. This harmless and
painless skin disorder can occur
on the arms, thighs, cheeks and
booty – it is usually caused by
nutritional deficiencies and it's
easy to fix

Triggers: nutritional deficiencies
including omega-3, beta-carotene/
vitamin A, biotin, pantothenic acid
and vitamin C

Foods to avoid: fatty meats rich in
saturated fat such as bacon and deli
meats, high omega-6 foods such
as cooking oils (favour extra virgin
olive oil for cooking), fried foods and
almonds

Food: eat 1 cup of beta-carotene rich
foods daily including sweet potato,
papaya and carrots; eat 1 cup of vitamin
C-rich foods daily including Brussels
sprouts, white potato, papaya and red
cabbage; eat 1 tsp of omega-3 – rich
flaxseeds and chia seeds or make Papaya
Flaxseed Drink (p. 116) or The Blue Healer
(p. 112) daily; see Menu 3 (p. 99).
Supplements: ½–1 tsp of flaxseed oil
or hemp seed oil daily (see omega-3
information, p. 64); biotin, pantothenic
acid and vitamin C (Skin Friend AM)

Leaky gut Cracks or holes in the gut allow toxins, bugs and partially digested food to penetrate into the tissues. Doctors call it 'increased intestinal permeability'; it can trigger inflammation and is associated with changes in gut flora and low vagal tone[2]	**Triggers:** alcohol, anxiety, aspirin (a salicylate medication), salicylate sensitivity, histamine intolerance, food allergies, poor diet, low fibre diets, excess sugar/sweetener, Candida albicans, overuse of antibiotics and some medical drugs, low vagal tone (Ch. 2), food poisoning and parasitic infection	**Food:** low histamine diet, lower salicylate intake and diagnose food intolerances; stimulate the vagus nerve (Ch. 2) **Supplements:** Skin Friend AM; omega-3 (see p. 64) Calm your nervous system (refer to vagal tone information in Ch. 2)
Light sensitivity, photophobia Intolerance to light sources including sunlight, fluorescent light and other artificial lighting Symptoms include itchy skin, headaches, sore eyes, eye problems and rashes that appear when light touches the skin and resolves quickly when away from light	**Triggers:** often linked to underlying anxiety disorders fear of sunlight, fear of skin cancer, fear of ageing, self-loathing, self-criticism of wrinkles and age spots (other causes include long-term use of topical corticosteroids)	**Food:** Menu 3 (p. 99), eat orange and purple foods daily, such as red cabbage, sweet potato and carrot. **Other:** In severe cases: DNRS brain retraining (see 'Helpful resources', p. 198), improve vagal tone (Ch. 2), daily gratitude

Mast cell activation syndrome (MCAS) Immune disorder with excess release of mast cells and inflammatory mediators such as histamine, which can cause allergic responses to foods, anaphylaxis, histamine intolerance, hives, eczema, swelling, low blood pressure, laboured breathing, rapid pulse, GIT symptoms, cold sensitivity. Can be linked to mould sickness (CIRS, p. 82) and autoimmune diseases	**Triggers:** overstimulated nervous system; high histamine diet; dysbiosis in microbiome – unhealthy microbes releasing high histamine; stress, trauma, negative beliefs, anxiety and other mood disorders, DAO enzyme deficiency (usually caused by ageing, nutritional deficiencies and excess histamine in the body) Probiotics may worsen it (histamine-lowering probiotics may be okay)	**Food:** identify allergies; eat low histamine diet with leek and green spring onion; (low salicylate if necessary); drink The Blue Healer daily (p. 112); download free histamine food list from skinfriend.com (join newsletter to receive it); avoid mould **Supplements:** DAO supplement with meals (and at night to see if your gut microbiome is making histamine at night: if so, DAO will temporarily alleviate symptoms); or make your own DAO by sprouting mung beans (p. 34) and pea shoots (p. 33); 500 mg glutathione (reduced or liposomal, no flavourings) and ½ tsp hemp seed oil (omega-3, see p. 64). Sip 3L (6.3 pt) spring/filtered water daily. **Other:** avoid stress; calm the nervous system with vagus nerve exercises (Ch. 2); liposomal vitamin C (if tolerated); practise gratitude daily If symptoms are severe look at DNRS brain training (see 'Helpful resources', p. 198)
Pigmentation (uneven) Age spots, liver spots, melasma (pregnancy mask)	**Triggers:** ageing skin, liver deficient in glutathione, pregnancy, a lifetime of sun exposure on fair skin, can happen alongside an autoimmune disorder (which can cause low glutathione)	**Supplements:** 500 mg glutathione daily (p. 67). It takes at least 3 months to break down the pigment and supplementation needs to be daily and ongoing to be permanent **Skin care:** apply sunscreen daily such as Synergie Skin ÜberZinc (face and body)
Psoriasis Autoimmune skin disorder where increased skin cell turnover rate causes a build-up of skin that is scaly and red. Sometimes it's itchy and painful	**Triggers:** calcium deficiency (or calcium malabsorption, which could be caused by magnesium deficiency – see calcium information, p. 60), chemical intolerance (possibly histamine intolerance and salicylate intolerance), anxiety, stress, depression, smoking	**Food:** Papaya Flaxseed Drink (p. 116) and The Blue Healer (p. 112); See menus 3 and Menu 4 (p. 99–100) **Supplements:** 300 mg calcium and magnesium daily (Skin Friend PM); ½–1 tsp flaxseed oil or hemp seed oil (omega-3, see p. 64); biotin, low dose B vitamins, zinc, molybdenum (Skin Friend AM). **Skin care:** Skin Friend 24-Hour Rescue Balm, Skin Friend Oat and Zinc Bath Powder, check vagal tone (Ch. 2)

Red skin syndrome (RSS)

A temporary and debilitating condition, also known as topical steroid addiction, topical steroid withdrawal (TSW) or topical corticosteroid addiction

Symptoms include bright red skin (like sunburn), red 'sleeves' on arms and legs (while palms and feet remain normal colour), hypersensitive skin, elephant (wrinkly) skin, severe flaking of the skin, irritated eyes, oozing skin, shedding skin, feeling too hot or too cold, nerve pain, swollen lymph nodes, fluid retention, hair loss, insomnia, fatigue, depression, anxiety

Important: when suddenly stopping long-term (high strength) topical steroid use, adrenal suppression (adrenal crisis) and HPA axis suppression can occur which can be life-threatening, so please consult with a doctor first, and read 'How to safely withdrawal from topical steroids' at eczemalife.com

Triggers: ceasing the use of topical corticosteroids after years of misuse. Not everyone who applies topical steroids will end up with RSS. For example, intermittently using it on small areas of your body will not result in RSS. But applying it to large areas of the body, at increasing strengths, for years can result in RSS that can last for months or several years.[3]

Tests: increased nitric oxide in the blood can cause the excess redness seen in people with RSS, so sufferers should get nitric oxide levels checked by a doctor

Research to read:

The work of Dr Marvin Rapaport, Clinical Professor of Dermatology at UCLA, at red-skin-syndrome.com: www.eczemalife.com (search 'TSW debate'); RSS support group and information: www.itsan.org

RSS recovery can be a slow process that only time can truly heal so you need doctor support and monitoring along the way.

Getting medical support: if you want a letter to give to your doctor to explain what RSS is, head to Dr Rapaport's website www.red-skin-syndrome.com and click on the 'White Paper' tab. Keep looking until you find a doctor willing to help you (if you live in Australia contact my team via support@skinfriend.com for a list of local doctors)

Food: The Blue Healer (p. 112), Papaya Flaxseed Drink (p. 116); follow Menu 3 (p. 99) and Menu 4 (p. 100).

Supplements: take nitric oxide lowering nutrients vitamin B12 and taurine (get your doctor to check your B12 level as you don't need it if it's high); Skin Friend AM

For improving sleep: calcium and magnesium (Skin Friend PM) and meditate each night or whenever you feel itchy

Clothing: Soft bamboo and/or 100% cotton clothing and bedding

Skin care: Skin Friend 24-Hour Rescue Balm, Skin Friend Oat and Zinc Bath Powder, if you have hair loss read 'Alopecia' (p. 80)

Other: Practise daily gratitude and read vagal tone information (Ch. 2)

Rosacea

First appears as mild redness, a bit like sunburn, but it worsens over time thanks to enlarged blood vessels under the skin. People with rosacea may also develop pimples, thickened skin and, in severe cases, a bulbous nose. It can occur at any age but it's most common in middle-aged women who have a history of blushing

Triggers: long-term inactivity (not exercising daily), stress, alcohol consumption, linked to food intolerances especially amine/histamine intolerance, dairy intolerance and sometimes also salicylate intolerance

Foods to avoid: histamine-rich foods (see p. 85); harsh sunlight, overheating, hot beverages, spicy foods, hot baths, alcohol, anxiety, worry, stress, rushing

Exercise is most important for long-term reversal of rosacea: do gentle exercise daily in air-conditioning to help improve the health of your blood vessels; learn to relax with deep breathing and meditation; wear a wide brimmed hat when outside
Food: low histamine/amine diet (see Menu 4, p. 100)
Supplements: magnesium, zinc, biotin, vitamin C and low dose B vitamins (Skin Friend AM) – must be low dose (avoid regular multivitamins as B vitamins are fermented and usually far too high a dosage which can worsen symptoms) – and calcium if diet is lacking (Skin Friend PM)
Other: place a cold compress around your neck, Skin Friend 24-Hour Rescue Balm; read vagal tone information (Ch. 2)

Salicylate sensitivity

Salicylate intolerance
Chemical intolerance
Aspirin sensitivity

Salicylates are a group of natural chemicals produced by plants for protection. A normal healthy diet can contain up to 200 mg of salicylates. Associated with eczema, hives, behavioural issues, ADHD, migraines, IBS, psoriasis, arthritis, rosacea, MCAS and mould sickness

Triggers: frequent or high chemical exposures; frequent perfume use; chemicals in toiletries; frequent alcohol consumption; crop spraying; eczema; MCAS (p. 87), mould sickness/CIRS (p. 82); illness; fatty liver; poor liver detoxification of chemicals (common in babies under age two)

Food: low salicylate diet, recipes in this book are low to moderate in salicylates (moderate salicylate foods are denoted with an S symbol). Refer to the Eczema Diet Shopping Guide from skinfriend.com (use code DETOX101 during checkout to get this low salicylate guide for free) or sign up to my newsletter for a free salicylate food chart PDF
Supplements: biotin, magnesium, calcium, glycine, vitamin B6 and zinc to detoxify salicylates more effectively (Skin Friend AM and Skin Friend PM)

Wrinkles

Premature ageing

Triggers: normal ageing process, excess sun exposure, smoking, drinking alcohol, dehydration, poor diet

Essential: wear a hat when outdoors, apply sunscreen to hands and face daily
Food: Papaya Flaxseed Drink (p. 116); see Menu 2 (p. 98); drink 3L (6.3 pt) of filtered/spring water daily
Supplements: 500 mg glutathione daily, zinc, pyridoxyl-5-phosphate (P-5-P), molybdenum, magnesium and biotin (Skin Friend AM), and calcium

PART 4
Menus and recipes

*Oat and Leek Flat Bread
(p. 156) with Sweet Potato
Nourish Bowl (p. 169)*

Chapter 7
Helpful guidelines (read me before beginning)

Remember you can tailor your HSK program to suit you. If you are allergic or sensitive to a particular food, simply avoid it. When following the menus, you can substitute any meal with another HSK recipe, especially if you are vegan or have other specific dietary needs.

Snacks

Ideally keep your meal times within 7 a.m. to 7 p.m. (or another 12-hour period that fits your life) so you fast for 12 hours each night ... unless eating out with friends, then have fun. Refrain from snacking throughout the day in order to avoid over-feeding your microbiome. If you get low blood sugar you can make Hemp Protein Balls (p. 135) or Healthy Banana Bread (p. 138) for an energizing snack. Refer to the menus and the recipe section.

Coffee and tea

If you need coffee, favour organic decaf coffee (it is the low salicylate/chemical option) or have a *half-strength* coffee (no sugar) and refer to milk options on p. 92. I find half- or quarter-strength coffee tastes much nicer and does not need sweetener to mask the bitter taste. Remember that coffee/caffeine blocks DAO enzyme production so avoid regular coffee and tea if you have eczema or any kind of skin inflammation. If you need a cuppa, opt for decaf coffee (if tolerated) and Carob Tea — it's the best (p. 115).

Eating out

Once you learn how to eat the HSK way, feel free to go out and have a social meal with your friends, because community and connection are important for your health and mental wellbeing.

Here are some tips when eating out: avoid fast food and deep fried meals such as fish and chips and fried chicken. Pick a meal that includes lots of fresh vegies, served with grilled fish, lamb, legumes or chicken (or an occasional steak!). Ask the waiter, 'Can I have the sauce/dressing on the side?' (if any) or, better yet, completely avoid sauce consumption, which is where you usually find the skin-sabotaging sugar, dairy and oils.

Cooking oil options for your skin type

Look up your skin type to find the right cooking oil for you:

Acne or oily skin types: no cooking oil is best (water fry instead) or use a little extra virgin olive oil as it won't make your skin oilier. Coconut oil may be okay but best to limit it and avoid all other oils.

Eczema, psoriasis and other skin rashes: no cooking oil (water fry instead) or use rice bran oil and pure sunflower oil (check there is no antioxidant), as they are the low salicylate and low amine options that also boost skin hydration. Use in moderation only.

Dry skin types or ageing skin (**no rashes**): pure sunflower oil (no antioxidant) or rice bran oil are the first choices. Coconut oil and extra virgin olive oil may be suitable if you do not have eczema or skin inflammation (see also 'Normal skin types' below).

Normal skin types (**no skin inflammation**): coconut oil or extra virgin olive oil (they are high in salicylates and amines but if you do not have chemical intolerance they are good choices). Both of these oils burn easily as they have a low smoking point (the pan will billow smoke quite quickly) so if you need to use high heat opt for rice bran oil as it has a high smoking point, therefore it is safer to cook with.

» Paleo note: paleo oils are coconut oil and extra virgin olive oil and paleo milks are hemp milk, cashew milk and coconut milk.

» Vegan note: all mentioned oils (above) and milks (below) are vegan-friendly so refer to your skin type for your best options.

Milk options for your skin type

Plant-based milks are any type of milk that is not from an animal source. I do not recommend dairy products (from cows, goats or sheep etc.) for the following science-based reasons that are discussed in the *New England Journal of Medicine* article 'Milk and health': when you consume dairy products, whether from cows, sheep or goats, you are consuming animal hormones, including increased levels of estrogens and progestins from pregnant cows.[1] Dairy products are recommended for calcium intake and bone health but the countries that consume the highest amounts of dairy have the highest rate of hip fracture (indicating poor bone health).[2]

And farmed milk is extracted from cows that are pregnant most of the time they are milked and it's an inhumane way to treat animals. Luckily we have plant-based milks which are yummy and good for us. Here are the HSK milk options for specific skin types:

Oat milk

It's cheap to buy, vegan-friendly, low salicylate and low amine, making it a good low chemical option. The natural beta-glucan in oat milk helps to lower cholesterol and trigger the satiety response (so you are less likely to overeat!). Note it contains a protein similar to gluten.

Tips: Shake the container before each use to make it creamy (as it settles on the bottom of the container when stored); buy unsweetened and check other ingredients before purchase (sunflower oil, water, salt and calcium are all good basic ingredients). If you can't find it in store, refer to the Creamy Oat Milk recipe (p. 42).

Cashew milk

It's vegan-friendly, low salicylate, low amine (but histamine producing), gluten-free and *much* nicer than almond milk. Shake the container before each use to make the cashew milk creamy. Available from supermarkets and health food shops, but check the other ingredients before purchase. Buy unsweetened as this milk already tastes great. You can also make your own (see p. 111)

Hemp milk

It's vegan-friendly, paleo-friendly and gluten-free (the level of salicylates and amines is unknown). Favour unsweetened (but note it's an acquired taste).

Rice milk

It's vegan-friendly, low salicylate, low amine and gluten-free. If you can't drink oat milk or cashew milk but need to avoid salicylates, then rice milk is your best option. Buy unsweetened as rice milk is already sweet.

Coconut water

Look, I don't love this option as coconut water is super rich in natural sugars and it's also very high in salicylates and amines so it's not suitable for people with eczema, skin inflammation or chemical intolerances. However, it's vegan-friendly, paleo-friendly and gluten-free so it could be the best option for some people. Favour unsweetened as coconut water is already super sweet. Coconut water may cause bloating in some people due to the high sugar content and it's not suitable for people with Candida albicans infections.

The healthy fish list

Choose any small white fish that is freshly caught (i.e. bought from a co-op, fish market or seafood shop, not a supermarket) such as flathead, dory, hake, flounder, sole or haddock. (Omega-3-rich fish include sardines, trout, rainbow trout and salmon — note that they contain high salicylates and high amines so they are not suitable if you are following Menu 4, see p. 100)

Fish to avoid

Big fish, higher up the food chain, contain higher levels of mercury, which can adversely affect brain health, so the following mercury-rich fish are not a part of the HSK program: flake/shark, marlin, swordfish, king mackerel, gulf tilefish, orange roughy, barramundi, gemfish, ling and fresh tuna (canned tuna is sourced from small fish so it's okay in moderation). If you eat high-mercury fish avoid all other seafood for at least two weeks and take mercury-detoxifying nutrients daily, including 500 mg glutathione (p. 67) and vitamin C (p. 53).

Salt options

In the recipes I mention using 'quality sea salt'. Best choices include natural sea salt, pink Himalayan salt (a type of rock salt), Celtic sea salt, natural iodized sea salt which has the added goodness of iodine for thyroid health (iodine is especially important during pregnancy) and rock salts such as Sendha Namak.

Check the ingredients before purchasing any type of salt. Do not consume salt that contains anti-caking agent (554) as it usually contains aluminium (read the fine print on the label). Do not consume regular table salt, which is highly refined and has anti-caking agent in it.

Alcohol and special occasions

Ideally abstain from drinking alcohol, especially when you are healing a skin disorder. If you want to drink alcohol on a special occasion, opt for the lower histamine/salicylate varieties — which are vodka and gin mixed with mineral water, or whiskey and water — as they are less likely to cause a hangover or adverse reactions. Do not drink more than three per night, and no more than once a week — alcohol is not good for your skin full stop (but having a social life is). Before bed, drink a large glass of water with a pinch of salt mixed in to rehydrate your body overnight.

Super hydrate

Your body is more than 60 per cent water (some estimate it's closer to 75 per cent) and, like a pot plant on grandma's balcony, you need to be watered daily or you will wrinkle and eventually die. Your body also needs an abundant supply of water to heal itself. If you have a skin problem (or three), whatever therapy or remedy you try could fail until you super hydrate your body. I call it 'super hydrate' because most of us falsely believe we are drinking enough … but optimal hydration is the goal here, and most of us miss the mark.

» If you suffer from dry skin, increased water intake can improve the skin's softness, smoothness and hydration, almost as much as a basic skin cream can.[3]

» A month of drinking 2 litres (4.2 pt) of water daily significantly boosts skin hydration in people who are not already big water drinkers.[4]

» Consuming enough water helps to relieve or prevent hangovers, migraines, angina, arthritis, asthma, colitis and high blood pressure according to Dr Batmanhelidj, author of *Your Body's Many Cries for Water*. I'm not suggesting you throw away your medications, but drink more water and see how good your body can feel.

How much water is enough?

If you are an adult, you need to drink at least 2 litres (4.2 pt) of water each day, or 3 litres (6.3 pt) of water if you exercised that day. To calculate how much water a teenager or a child should drink, multiply their weight (in kilograms) by 0.033 to work out how many litres. If using pounds, halve their weight to calculate how many fluid ounces of water. For example, 110 lbs ÷ 2 = 55 fl oz water.

Water drinking tips

» Buy a 1.5 litre (3 pt) water bottle and each day fill it with filtered or spring water. Add two or three pinches of quality sea salt to help the water penetrate into your cells where it's needed most. Don't add too much salt as it should be pleasant to drink!

» To prevent bacteria growth over time, each night wash the water bottle in hot, soapy water and then rinse with fresh water before refilling it.

» I use a Brita filter jug and replace the filter every eight weeks — the jug needs to be washed in soapy hot water every eight weeks.

» I also buy natural spring water from my local organic food market each week — it's convenient for me, but drink whatever is available to you … Filtered tap water is better than drinking nothing and being dehydrated!

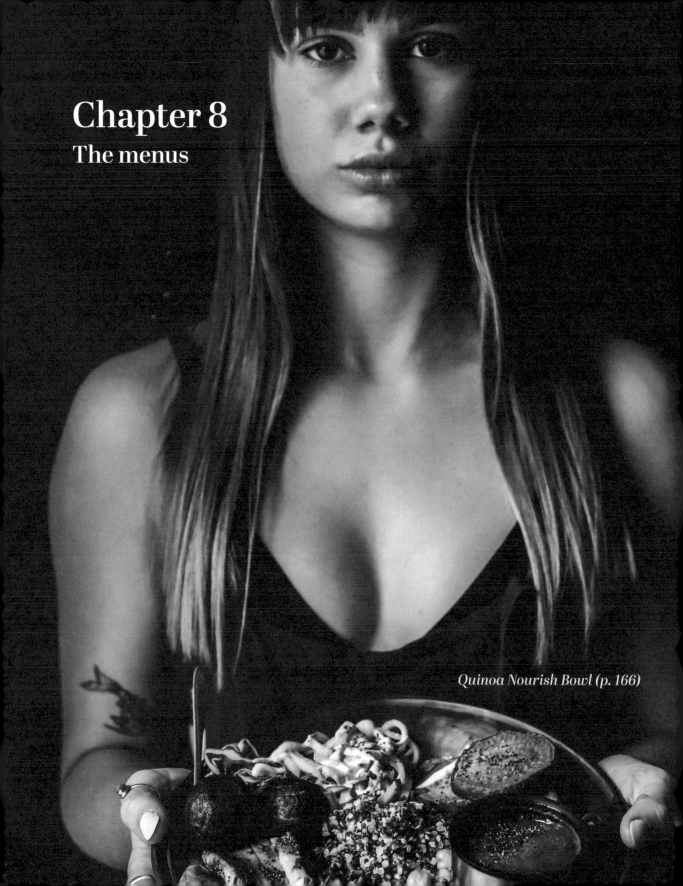

Chapter 8
The menus

Quinoa Nourish Bowl (p. 166)

Menu 1: Clear skin

This menu is ideal for people with oily skin, pimples or acne. Note you can tailor this menu to suit you by choosing any of the meals on this menu, in any order you like.

Breakfast	Lunch	Dinner
DAO Smoothie (p. 109) and/or Overnight Oats (p. 119) – make two and have one tomorrow	Sweet Potato Boats (p. 180) – make six to consume throughout the week (eat two halves per serving)	Healthy Fish Tacos (p. 187) or San Choy Bau (p. 159)
DAO Smoothie (p. 109) and/or Overnight Oats (p. 119) or Banana Flour Pancakes (p. 195)	Sweet Potato Boats (p. 180)	Lamb Skewers (p. 164) with leftover Sweet Potato Boats (p. 180)
DAO Smoothie (p. 109) and/or Papaya Beauty Smoothie Bowl (p. 126) – make two and have one tomorrow	Creamy Oat and Vegetable Soup (p. 177)	Creamy Oat and Vegetable Soup (p. 177)
Papaya Beauty Smoothie Bowl (p. 126) and/or Healthy Skin Juice (p. 116)	Sweet Potato Nourish Bowl (p. 169) or Cashew Caesar Salad (p. 170), make enough for tomorrow's lunch	Lamb and Zucchini Pasta (p. 183)
Banana Beet Smoothie (p. 110) and/or Sweet Potato Toast (p. 123)	Sweet Potato Nourish Bowl (p. 169) or Cashew Caesar Salad (p. 170)	Green Detox Soup (p. 179) or Beet Detox Soup (p. 149), make the roasted chickpeas (garbanzo beans) or black beans with no oil or use extra virgin olive oil
Papaya Sunrise Porridge (p. 120) or DAO Smoothie (p. 109)	Leftover Green Detox Soup (p. 179) or Quinoa Nourish Bowl (p. 166) with chicken	Leftovers or Sweet Potato Flatbread (p. 150) with San Choy Bau (p. 159)
Banana Beet Smoothie (p. 110) or Healthy Skin Juice (p. 116) and/ or Banana Flour Pancakes or Oat Crepes (no oil) (p. 195)	Leftover Sweet Potato Flatbread (p. 150) with lean chicken or lamb, red cabbage and leeks	Asparagus and Black Bean Soft Tacos (p. 155)

Acne-friendly snacks and treats include: Banana Beet Nice Cream (p. 188), Pink Pear Sorbet (p. 196), Healthy Banana Bread (p. 138), herbal teas (no sweetener), Carob Tea (p. 115), fresh vegetable juices (limit fruit), Healthy Skin Juice (p. 116), DAO Smoothie (p. 109) or any of the smoothie recipes.*

*Remember: don't add any oils or seeds including hemp seed oil, chia or flaxseed as they could make your skin oilier.

Menu 2: Firm and tone

This menu is ideal for people with cellulite, wrinkles, keratosis pilaris and ageing skin. Sweeteners are generally ageing on the skin but a little stevia, maple syrup or rice malt syrup is okay in moderation (rice syrup is alkalizing and fructose-free). If you are hungry, snack on carrot and celery sticks with Beetroot Hummus (p. 145) or Carrot Dip (p. 145) or Hemp Protein Balls (p. 135). Sip 3 litres (6.3 pt) of water throughout the day. Refer to Chapter 7 for oil and milk options for your skin type and tips on eating out. Note you can tailor this menu to suit you by choosing any of the meals on this menu, in any order you like.

Breakfast	Lunch	Dinner
(pre-freeze papaya) Papaya Flaxseed Drink (p. 116) and/or Sweet Potato Toast (p. 123)	Sweet Potato Boats (p. 180) with chicken or fish – make six boats for throughout the week (eat two halves per serving) but cook the meat fresh each day	Beet Detox Soup (p. 149) or San Choy Bau (p. 159)
The Blue Healer (p. 112) and/or Overnight Oats (p. 119)	Sweet Potato Boats (p. 180) or leftover Beet Detox Soup (p. 149)	Crispy Chicken (p. 184) with Vegan Mayo (p. 146) or leftover Beet Detox Soup (p. 149)
Cabbage Steaks with Beet Cream (p. 125)	Sweet Potato Boats (p. 180) or leftover Beet Detox Soup (p. 149)	Lamb Skewers (p. 164) with leftover Sweet Potato Boats (p. 180) or Sweet Potato Nourish Bowl (p. 169)
(pre-freeze papaya) Papaya Flaxseed Drink (p. 116) and/or Sweet Potato Toast (p. 123)	Cashew Caesar Salad (p. 170) – make two and have one tomorrow	Healthy Fish Tacos (p. 187)
Papaya Beauty Smoothie Bowl (p. 126) or Hemp Protein Balls (p. 135)	Leftover Cashew Caesar Salad (p. 170)	Asparagus and Black Bean Soft Tacos (p. 155)
Papaya Sunrise Porridge (p. 120) or Overnight Oats (p. 119)	Green Detox Soup (p. 179)	Sweet Potato Nourish Bowl (p. 169)
Cabbage Steaks with Beet Cream (p. 125) and/or DAO Smoothie (p. 109)	Leftover Green Detox Soup (p. 179)	Lamb and Zucchini Pasta (p. 183)

Snacks and treats include: Banana Beet Nice Cream (p. 188), Pink Pear Sorbet (p. 196), Hemp Protein Balls (p. 135), herbal teas (no sweetener), Carob Tea (p. 115), fresh vegetable juices (limit or no fruit), Healthy Skin Juice (p. 116), DAO Smoothie (p. 109) or any of the smoothie recipes.

Menu 3: Nourish/detox

This menu is for anyone who wants to nourish their skin, detox and promote immune wellness. It's also suitable for people with dry skin and skin inflammation such as eczema, dermatitis, psoriasis, rosacea, red skin syndrome, dandruff and keratosis pilaris. Note you can tailor this menu to suit you by choosing any of the meals on this menu, in any order you like.

Breakfast	Lunch	Dinner
DAO Smoothie (p. 109) and/or Banana Bliss Overnight Oats (p. 120) – make two (minus the topping) and have one tomorrow	Sweet Potato Boats (p. 180) – make six to consume throughout the week (eat two halves per serving) and Roasted Maple Brussel Bites (p. 132)	Quinoa Nourish Bowl (p. 166) with leftover Sweet Potato Boats (p. 180) or Quinoa and Chicken Salad with Beet Cream (p. 163)
The Blue Healer (p. 112) and/or Banana Bliss Overnight Oats (p. 120) or Cabbage Steaks with Beet Cream (p. 125)	Leftovers (always cook meats fresh) or Hemp Protein Balls (p. 135)	Lamb Skewers (p. 164) with leftover Sweet Potato Boats (p. 180) or Cabbage Steaks with Beet Cream (p. 125)
Sweet Potato Toast (p. 123) or Golden Crunch Granola (p. 129) with Healthy Skin Juice (p. 116)	Beet Detox Soup (p. 149) or Cashew Caesar Salad (p. 170); replace cashews with chickpeas (garbanzo beans) if needed	Beet Detox Soup (p. 149) or Crispy Sweet Potato Gnocchi (p. 174) with Roasted Maple Brussel Bites (p. 132)
Papaya Beauty Smoothie Bowl (p. 126) – make two and have one tomorrow; or 3 x Carob and Flax Protein Balls (p. 136) and Healthy Skin Juice (p. 116)	Sweet Potato Nourish Bowl (p. 169) or Cashew Caesar Salad (p. 170); make two and have one tomorrow, but cook meat fresh each day	Healthy Fish Tacos (p. 187) Optional extras: Roasted Maple Brussel Bites (p. 132) or Charred Cos Lettuce (p. 173) or Creamy Oat and Vegetable Soup (p. 177)
Papaya Beauty Smoothie Bowl (p. 126) and/or The Blue Healer (p. 112) or Carob Smoothie (p. 110)	Sweet Potato Nourish Bowl (p. 169) or Cashew Caesar Salad (p. 170) (swap cashews for chickpeas/ garbanzo beans if needed)	Green Detox Soup (p. 179) or Creamy Oat and Vegetable Soup (p. 173)
Cabbage Steaks with Beet Cream (p. 125) or Golden Granola (p. 129) and DAO Smoothie (p. 109)	Leftovers such as Green Detox Soup (p. 179) or Creamy Oat and Vegetable Soup (p. 177) (cook your meat fresh daily) or Cashew Caesar Salad (p. 170)	Crispy Chicken (p. 184) with Charred Cos Lettuce (p. 173) or Crispy Sweet Potato Gnocchi (p. 174) with Roasted Maple Brussel Bites (p. 132)
Papaya Flaxseed Drink (p. 116) and 3 x Carob and Flax Protein Balls (p. 136) or Oat Crepes (p. 195)	Sweet Potato Flatbread (p. 150) with San Choy Bau (p. 159) or Cashew Caesar Salad (p. 170)	Asparagus and Black Bean Soft Tacos (p. 155) or Lamb and Zucchini Pasta (p. 183)

Snacks and treats include: Banana Beet Nice Cream (p. 188), Pink Pear Sorbet (p. 196), Hemp Protein Balls (p. 135), Healthy Banana Bread (p. 138), Carob Tea (p. 115), Healthy Skin Juice (p. 116), DAO Smoothie (p. 109) or any of the smoothie recipes.

Menu 4: Low histamine/salicylate

I used this menu when I had severe histamine intolerance and salicylate intolerance. This way of eating stopped the itch — quickly clearing half of my symptoms — and made life bearable, which is the only reason I am sharing it with the (very) few people who will actually need it. Menu 4 is to be used in conjunction with calming your nervous system and creating an inner sanctuary (see Chapter 2). Begin on Menu 4 and progress to Menu 3, and get professional advice and support along the way. Important:

» If you are a child, underweight, going through red skin syndrome (RSS), very ill, pregnant or breastfeeding this menu is *not* for you.

» You need to take supplements while following this menu (refer to The Blue Healer recipe for the supplements, on p. 112).

» If you already know you adversely react to a food on this menu, simply avoid this food and sub it with one you can safely eat. If you are sensitive to oats try quinoa, which can be boiled in water and made into porridge etc.

» Only eat when you are happy and relaxed — laughing while you eat helps your body to accept foods better (so avoid watching the news or thrillers during this time).

» Avoid using cashews in these recipes as all nuts produce histamines, and avoid potato if needed (you can test potato, if desired, after a couple of weeks — I ate it on treat days).

» Eat as much as you like on this menu — don't go hungry.

» Remember to cook your meat fresh each day (as cooked meats develop amines overnight), and use up leftovers such as flatbreads within three to four days.

» If you are highly sensitive to salicylates avoid sweet potato on treat days (as it's moderate in salicylates).

» Listen to calming music, such as my own Vagus Nerve Wellness Playlist, when you eat to switch your nervous system into 'rest and digest' mode (refer to 'Helpful resources', p. 198).

Cooking oils

You are probably best to avoid all cooking oils until your symptoms are under control. If needed, rice bran oil and sunflower oil are low in both salicylates and amines so they may be an option for you — I was okay with a little sunflower oil. To keep your skin soft and hydrated, consume ½ teaspoon of either hemp seed oil or flaxseed oil daily (increase this to 1 teaspoon or more during winter) — this is important (try The Blue Healer, p. 112).

Sweeteners

Sweeteners are generally bad for inflammation, Candida albicans and gut microbiome issues. While on this menu, ideally avoid using sweeteners or refer to Menu 4 Snacks and treats (opposite) for special occasions.

Breakfast	Lunch	Dinner
The Blue Healer (p. 112) and Overnight Oats (p. 119); make two and have one tomorrow or as an afternoon snack	Cashew Caesar Salad (p. 170) with sliced organic chicken thigh, iceberg lettuce, mung bean sprouts and red cabbage (no dressing, cos/romaine or cashews)	San Choy Bau (p. 159) with organic beef mince Optional: Oat and Leek Flatbread (p. 156) or use iceberg lettuce leaf cups
The Blue Healer (p. 112) and Overnight Oats (p. 119)	San Choy Bau (p. 159) with organic chicken mince or thigh fillets Optional: Oat and Leek Flatbread (p. 156) or use iceberg lettuce leaf cups	Creamy Oat and Vegetable Soup (p. 177) with organic chicken thigh fillets or organic fresh mince
The Blue Healer (p. 112) with glutathione and Papaya Sunrise Porridge (p. 120) – with pear or no fruit; avoid papaya if you have amine intolerance	San Choy Bau (p. 159) Optional: Oat and Leek Flatbread (p. 156) or use iceberg lettuce leaf cups	Lamb Skewers (p. 164) with water fried red cabbage, leeks and green spring onions/shallots/scallions (no zucchini if you are salicylate intolerant)
The Blue Healer (p. 112) and Oat Crepes (p. 195) or Overnight Oats (p. 119)	Cashew Caesar Salad (p. 170) with sliced organic chicken thigh, iceberg lettuce, mung bean sprouts and red cabbage (no dressing or cashews; no cos/romaine lettuce if you are highly salicylate intolerant)	Crispy Chicken (p. 184) with optional White Bean Sauce (p. 146); note some people with severe histamine intolerance can't eat beans/legumes
The Blue Healer (p. 112) and Overnight Oats (p. 119)	San Choy Bau (p. 159) Optional: Oat and Leek Flatbread (p. 156) or use iceberg lettuce cups	Creamy Oat and Vegetable Soup (p. 177)
The Blue Healer (p. 112) and Overnight Oats (p. 119)	Cashew Caesar Salad (p. 170) with iceberg lettuce, mung bean sprouts and red cabbage (no dressing, cos/romaine or cashews)	San Choy Bau (p. 159) Optional: Oat and Leek Flatbread (p. 156) or use iceberg lettuce leaf cups
The Blue Healer (p. 112) and Oat and Leek Flatbread (p. 156) or Overnight Oats (p. 119)	San Choy Bau (p. 159) Optional: Oak and Leek Flatbread (p. 156) or use iceberg lettuce leaf cups	If you can eat fish ... Healthy Fish Tacos (p. 187) with iceberg lettuce (quick GF option) or Oat and Leek Flatbread (p. 156) or Soft Tacos (p. 153). Take a DAO supplement if needed or substitute the fish with black beans, beef mince or chicken.

Snacks and treats include: If you are hungry here are some healthy options: make extra batches of Overnight Oats (p. 119) – oats are great for promoting satiety and a good night's sleep; Pink Pear Sorbet *without the beetroot* (p. 196), Oat Bliss Balls (p. 135) and Saffron Tea (p. 115). Avoid these snacks in weeks 1 and 2, to see how your body responds to the menu in pure form. Special occasions and eating out: refer to Menu 3 (p. 99) and if you have histamine intolerance take a DAO supplement or make the DAO Smoothie (p. 109) and drink it with meals. My favourite treat meals were roast potatoes (homemade) and a burger on a gluten-free bun with plain grilled chicken and iceberg lettuce.

Menu 5: Vegan

Mix it up or follow this menu in order and then choose your favourites for the following week.

Breakfast	Lunch	Dinner
DAO Smoothie (p. 109) and/or Overnight Oats (p. 119) – make two (minus the topping) and have one tomorrow	Sweet Potato Boats (p. 180) – make six to consume throughout the week (eat two halves per serving) with Roasted Black Beans (p. 149)	Quinoa Nourish Bowl (p. 166) with leftover Sweet Potato Boats (p. 180)
The Blue Healer (p. 112) and/or Banana Bliss Overnight Oats (p. 120)	Leftovers or Quinoa Nourish Bowl (p. 166)	Cabbage Steaks with Beet Cream (p. 125)
Sweet Potato Toast (p. 123) with Healthy Skin Juice (p. 116)	Beet Detox Soup (p. 149) with Roasted Black Beans (p. 131), make enough for a second meal tonight	Beet Detox Soup (p. 149) with Roasted Black Beans (p. 131)
Papaya Beauty Smoothie Bowl (p. 126) – make two and have one tomorrow; or 3 x Carob and Flax Protein Balls (p. 136) and Healthy Skin Juice (p. 116)	Sweet Potato Nourish Bowl (p. 169), make two and have one tomorrow	Cashew Caesar Salad (p. 170) with Roasted Chickpeas (p. 131) and Cashew Cream (p. 142)
Papaya Beauty Smoothie Bowl (p. 126) and/or The Blue Healer (p. 112) or Carob Smoothie (p. 110)	Leftover Sweet Potato Nourish Bowl (p. 169) or Cashew Caesar Salad (p. 170)	Green Detox Soup (p. 179) or Sweet Potato Flatbread (p. 150) with Cashew Caesar Salad (p. 170)
Cabbage Steaks with Beet Cream (p. 125) or Golden Granola (p. 129) and DAO Smoothie (p. 109)	Leftovers such as Green Detox Soup (p. 179) or Creamy Oat and Vegetable Soup (p. 177)	Crispy Sweet Potato Gnocchi (p. 174) with Roasted Maple Brussel Bites (p. 132)
Papaya Flaxseed Drink (p. 116) and/or Golden Granola (p. 129) or Oat Crepes (p. 195)	Leftover Sweet Potato Flatbread (p. 150) with San Choy Bau (p. 159) with chickpeas (garbanzo beans)	Asparagus and Black Bean Soft Tacos (p. 155)

Snacks and treats include: All of the desserts are vegan; see pp. 188–97 for options or snack on Healthy Banana Bread (p. 138), Carob Tea (p. 115) and any of the yummy protein balls (pp. 135–36) and dips (p. 145).

Menu 6: Paleo/immune wellness

Mix it up or follow this menu in order and then choose your favourites for the following week.
If you have histamine intolerance avoid cashews in the recipes.

Breakfast	Lunch	Dinner
DAO Smoothie (p. 109) and/or Sweet Potato Toast (p. 123)	Cashew Caesar Salad (p. 170) with sliced organic chicken thigh	San Choy Bau (p. 159) with organic beef mince in iceberg lettuce leaf cups
The Blue Healer (p. 112) with hemp milk or cashew milk (or milk to suit your skin type) and Banana Flour Pancakes (p. 195) with hemp milk	Sweet Potato Boats (p. 180) with organic beef mince	Crispy Chicken (p. 184) (no oat flour, no vegan mayo) with zucchini pasta (p. 183) or leftover sweet potato
The Blue Healer (p. 112) with hemp milk (or milk to suit your skin type) and/or Cabbage Steaks and Beet Cream (p. 125)	Sweet Potato Boats (p. 180) with organic chicken mince (or meat of choice) and Charred Cos Lettuce (p. 173)	Beet Detox Soup (p. 149), omit the beans (replace with cooked beef mince if desired)
DAO Smoothie (p. 109) and/or Sweet Potato Toast (p. 123)	Leftover Beet Detox Soup (p. 149)	Sweet Potato Nourish Bowl (p. 169) with organic chicken
Papaya Beauty Smoothie Bowl (p. 126), make two and have one tomorrow	San Choy Bau (p. 159) served in lettuce leaf cups	Crispy Sweet Potato Gnocchi (p. 174) or Lamb and Zucchini Pasta (p. 183)
Papaya Beauty Smoothie Bowl (p. 126)	Cashew Caesar Salad (p. 170)	Healthy Fish Tacos (p. 187) served in cos or iceberg lettuce cups
DAO Smoothie (p. 109) Roasted Maple Brussel Bites (p. 132) or Cabbage Steaks and Beet Cream (p. 125)	Beet Detox Soup (p. 149), omit the beans	Lamb Skewers (p. 164) with Roasted Maple Brussel Bites (p. 132)

Snacks and treats include: Banana Beet Nice Cream (p. 188) with hemp milk, Pink Pear Sorbet (p. 196), Saffron Tea (p. 115) with hemp milk, and Banana Flour Pancakes (p. 195) with hemp milk or cashew milk.

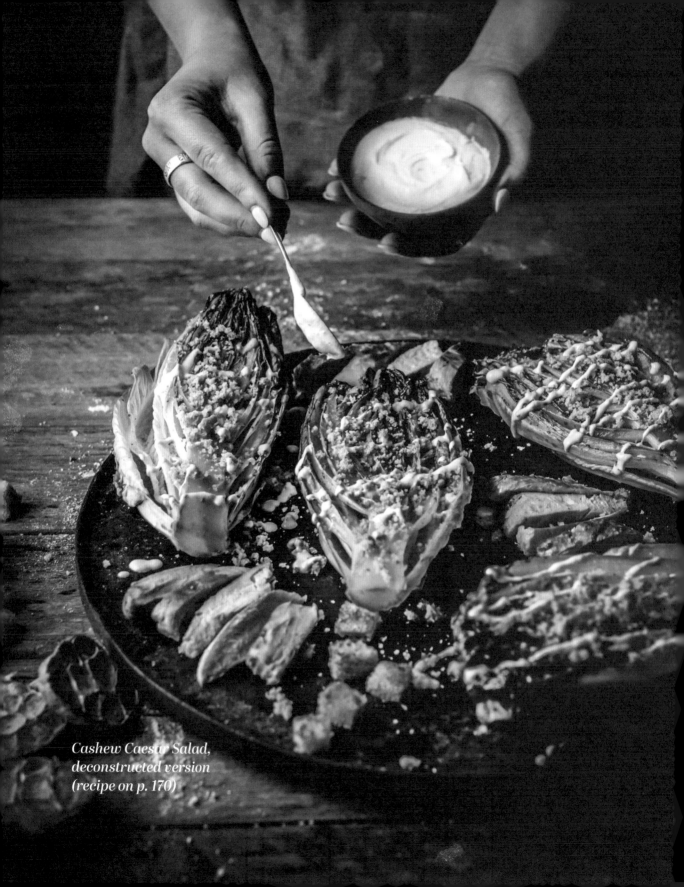

*Cashew Caesar Salad,
deconstructed version
(recipe on p. 170)*

Chapter 9
Healthy Skin Kitchen recipes

Recipes by Karen Fischer and Katie Layland

I have always prized cookbooks, diets and health books by the quality of their recipes. I have often thought: sure, it's easy to make meals appear yummy with cups of sugar, butter, bacon and chorizo sausage but these 'go-to' ingredients don't induce glowing skin or good heart health. Skip the first hundred pages of spiel in any diet or health book and flip to the back — to the recipe section — and you will see how doable the diet is. Many health experts buy recipes for their books or overly rely on pimple-promoting almonds, dates and cacao to make everything taste good, and some don't have recipes at all because it's not easy to design good grub. The following recipes have been developed, tested and tweaked (a lot!) until my family and I loved them. Many of these recipes are my mainstay — an essential part of my daily routine so I can feel great and have glowing good health. Nutritionist Katie Layland, who has worked at my office for years and knows my programs by heart, helped to create extra recipes so we could give you plenty of variety, flavours and meal plans. We have cut down on the salt, swapped the sugar and increased the vegetable content — even adding them to smoothies and flatbreads! — until I was happy with the health benefits and the flavours. I hope you love them as much as we do.

Symbols and their meanings

You will find these symbols beside specific ingredients within the recipes:

(H) avoid this food if you are histamine intolerant

(A) moderate source of amines

(AA) rich source of amines

(S) moderate source of salicylates

(GF) Gluten-free

(G) Contains gluten

Symbols

You will find these symbols above the recipes:

a	moderate source of amines
aa	rich source of amines
fid	Food Intolerance Diagnosis (FID) Program: low salicylate and low histamine recipe or option
gf	gluten-free recipe
gfo	recipe has a gluten-free option
M4	Menu 4: low salicylate and low histamine recipe or option
pal	recipe is paleo-friendly or has a paleo option
s	moderate source of salicylates
ss	rich source of salicylates
veg	vegetarian and vegan-friendly or has a vegan option

What is the FID Program?

In the recipes you will see that I sometimes mention the FID Program. The Food Intolerance Diagnosis (or FID) Program features in my book *The Eczema Detox*. It is a low salicylate, low amine diagnostic program and is designed to be restrictive for the first fourteen days to help you work out which foods are triggering your skin problems — it's basically the same as Menu 4, so if you are new to the FID Program all you need to do is follow Menu 4 in this book.

Volume equivalents

Metric	Imperial (approximate)
20 ml	½ fl oz
60 ml	2 fl oz
80 ml	3 fl oz
125 ml	4½ fl oz
160 ml	5½ fl oz
180 ml	6 fl oz
250 ml (1 cup)	9 fl oz
375 ml	13 fl oz
500 ml	18 fl oz
750 ml	27 fl oz
1 L	25 fl oz

Weight equivalents

Metric	Imperial (approximate)
10 g	⅓ oz
50 g	2 oz
80 g	3 oz
100 g	3½ oz
150 g	5 oz
175 g	6 oz
200 g	7 oz
250 g	9 oz
375 g	13 oz
400 g	14 oz
500 g	1 lb
750 g	1 lb 10 oz
1 kg	2 lb

Oven temperatures

°Celsius (C)	°Fahrenheit (F)
120	235
150	300
180	350
200	400
220	425

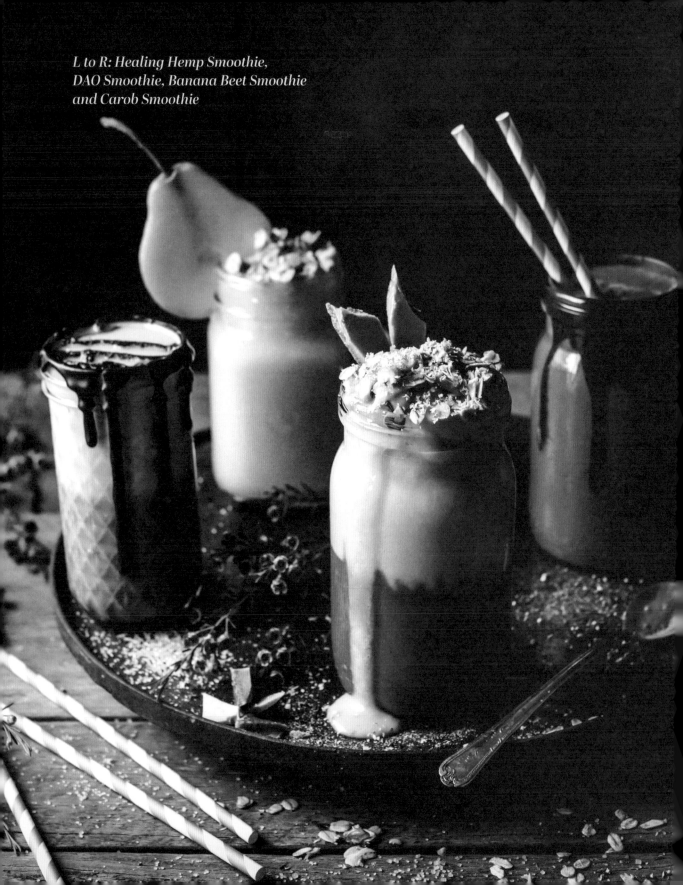

L to R: Healing Hemp Smoothie,
DAO Smoothie, Banana Beet Smoothie
and Carob Smoothie

Chapter 10
Drinks

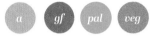

Healing Hemp Smoothie

Serves 1, preparation time 3 minutes, pre-freeze fruit if desired

Fix dry skin, hair loss and weak nails with the Healing Hemp Smoothie, which is an excellent source of skin-hydrating omega-3 oils and protein to strengthen hair and nails. We decorated this smoothie with Carob Mylk Chocolate Bar mixture (p. 192).

- 1½–2 cups plant-based milk of choice (see p. 92)
- ¼ cup hemp protein powder (plain, not flavoured)
- ½ banana (A) or ½ peeled pear (pre-sliced and frozen)
- 4 ice cubes

Place all the ingredients into a high-speed blender and blend on high until smooth.

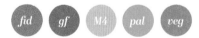

DAO Smoothie

Serves 1, preparation time 6 minutes, pre-freeze pear if desired

Cleanse your digestive system and reduce histamines for gorgeous gut wellness with this refreshing smoothie, rich in plant-based sprout DAO. The pulverizing action of the blender releases the DAO, making it readily available. If you would like to grow your own sprouts, refer to 'How to sprout pea shoots' (p. 33) or 'How to sprout mung beans' (p. 34). If you have acne, psoriasis, rosacea or eczema add Skin Friend AM.

- ¼ cup celery, washed, strings removed, then finely sliced
- 1 small handful pea shoots or mung bean sprouts, washed
- ½ large pear, peeled, core removed, then diced (pre-frozen)
- ½ cup filtered or spring water
- 4 ice cubes
- 2 scoops Skin Friend AM (optional)

Place all the ingredients into a high-speed blender and blend on high until smooth.

Banana Beet Smoothie

Makes 1 large serving, preparation time 10 minutes, pre-freeze fruit overnight

Go all pink or half and half, with alkalizing beetroot to give your skin a healthy glow. If you have acne or eczema add Skin Friend AM.

- ½–1 banana (A; sliced and pre-frozen overnight)
- 2 cups plant-based milk of choice (see p. 92)
- ¼ cup plant protein powder of choice (such as pea protein)
- 5 ice cubes
- 1–2 tablespoons grated fresh beetroot/beet (peeled) (S)

Place the banana, milk, protein powder and ice cubes into a high-speed blender and blend until smooth. Pour half of the mixture into a jar and place it into the freezer. To the second half of the mixture, add the beetroot and blend until smooth. Pour the beet mixture into a jar, then pour the banana smoothie on top. We decorated this smoothie with Golden Granola (p. 129).

Carob Smoothie

Serves 1, preparation time 5 minutes, pre-freeze fruit overnight (optional)

Enjoy this delicious low salicylate, low amine smoothie at any time of the day. If you are not on the FID Program, see p. 92 for other milk options.

- 1 peeled pear (cut into cubes and pre-frozen)
- 1 heaped tablespoon carob powder (roasted or raw)
- 1½ cups organic rice milk (GF option) or oat milk (contains gluten)
- ½ teaspoon hemp seed oil or flaxseed oil (begin on ¼ teaspoon)
- 1 teaspoon real maple syrup or brown rice syrup (optional)

Place all the ingredients into a high-speed blender and blend until smooth. We decorated this smoothie with Carob Mylk Chocolate Bar mixture (p. 192).

Cashew Milk

Makes 4 servings, preparation time 5 minutes plus soaking time

Creamy, tasty and nutritious — cashew milk is one of the best-tasting DIY milks (it's so much nicer than hemp or almond milk!). Cashews are a seed, not a nut, and a natural prebiotic that is good for your microbiome. I make cashew milk syrup-free and add electrolytes (calcium and magnesium) to support healthy bones and teeth and to improve my sleep. Soak the cashews in warm water for 4 to 8 hours to activate the cashews (do not soak for longer as they get too soft). Or for a quick batch, soak the cashews in boiling hot water for 30 minutes. Drain and rinse well.

- ¾ cup raw cashews, soaked (H)
- 5 cups filtered or spring water
- 3 scoops calcium and magnesium powder (Skin Friend PM)
- ½–1 teaspoon pure maple syrup (totally optional, taste it first)

Process the milk in batches if needed. Place half the cashews and half the water (2½ cups) into a high-speed blender and blend until smooth and creamy. If you are using a regular blender or food processor you might need to strain the milk with a milk bag, cheesecloth or fine strainer.

Do the second batch and add the syrup and calcium/magnesium powder, if using, and blend until smooth. Combine the two batches in a large jug, mix and store in the refrigerator for up to four days. Stir each time before using.

The Blue Healer

Serves 1, preparation time 5 minutes

My favourite skin saviour recipe for healing and repairing the skin. It's deliberately sweetener-free and fruit-free and surprisingly pleasant tasting, depending on the type of milk you use (I use organic unsweetened oat milk — shake your milk before using to disperse the creaminess). The supplements are optional, but note it's the magnesium glycinate and B vitamins in Skin Friend AM that change this naturally purple smoothie to aqua/blue. If you are following Menu 4 (p. 100) begin with ¼ teaspoon of hemp seed oil for a few days and favour oat milk or rice milk. If you would like to grow your own sprouts, refer to 'How to sprout pea shoots' (p. 33) and 'How to sprout mung beans' (p. 34). If you have MCAS or severe histamine intolerance, stir in 500 g of glutathione powder after you have finished blending (as high-speed blending can damage glutathione) or take in capsule form.

- 1 cup organic oat milk (contains gluten) or GF plant-based milk of choice (p. 92) or blend 1 cup filtered or spring water with ¼ cup rolled oats until smooth
- 1 tablespoon fresh mung bean sprouts or pea shoots, rinsed in water
- ¼ cup finely sliced red cabbage
- ½ teaspoon hemp seed oil or flaxseed oil (begin on ¼ teaspoon)
- 1 g magnesium glycinate/bisglycinate powder* and/or 2 scoops Skin Friend AM (optional)

Place all the ingredients in a high-speed blender and blend until smooth.

*1 g is about 125 mg of elemental magnesium in magnesium glycinate or magnesium bisglycinate powder (depending on the brand).

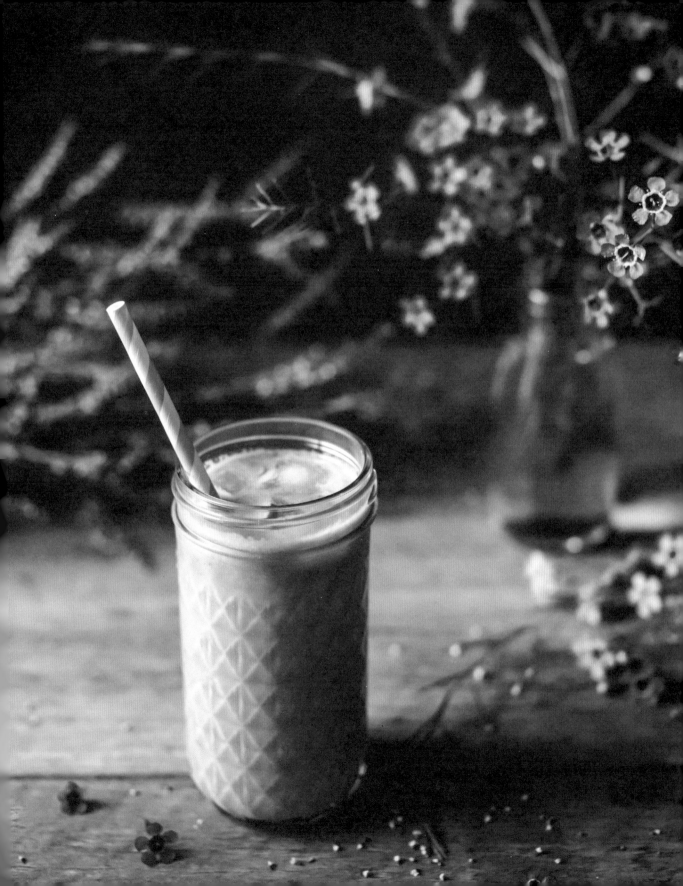

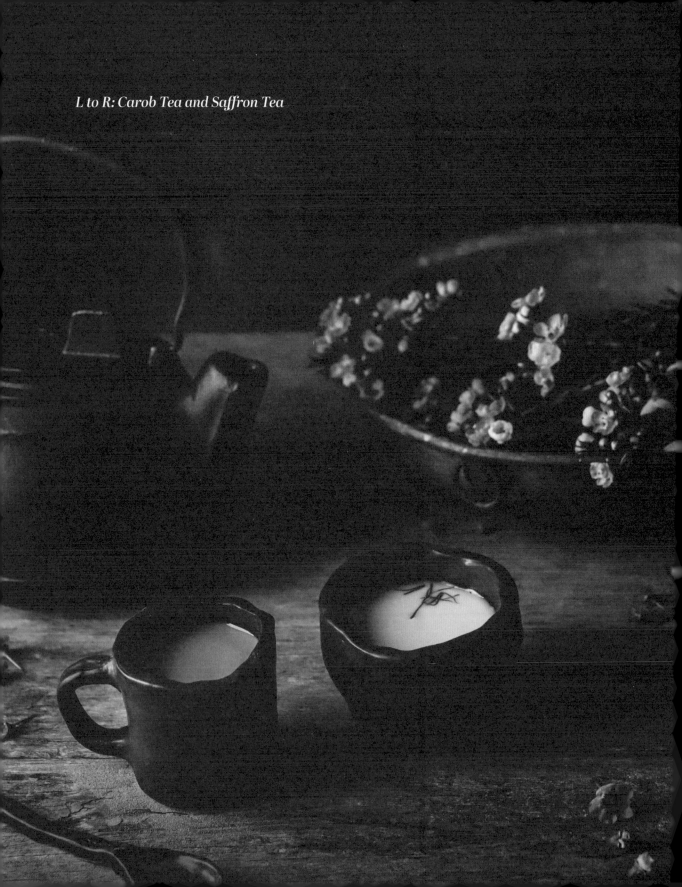

L to R: Carob Tea and Saffron Tea

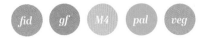

Carob Tea

Serves 1, preparation time 4 minutes

Sleep well with the combined calming effects of carob, calcium, magnesium and glycine, an amino acid and neurotransmitter that increases serotonin to improve sleep and mood, heals the gut and enables the production of collagen in the skin. I make this drink with oat milk and without sweetener, but you can add ½ teaspoon of rice malt syrup or real maple syrup if needed.

- 2 teaspoons carob powder (roasted or raw)
- 1–1½ cups plant-based milk of choice (p. 92)
- 2 scoops calcium and magnesium powder (Skin Friend PM, also contains glycine)

Pour a little boiling hot water into a tea/coffee cup (approximately 3 tablespoons). Add the carob powder and mix. Meanwhile, heat the milk in a small saucepan until it's warm, then pour it into the cup and mix well. Mix in calcium and magnesium powder if desired.

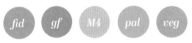

Saffron Tea

Serves 1, preparation time 10 minutes

Saffron has anti-inflammatory properties and contains safranal and crocin, which calms minor stomach disorders and soothes coughs.[1] Add calcium and magnesium powder to promote a good night's sleep (optional, of course).

- 1 cup plant-based milk of choice (p. 92)
- 3–4 small strands saffron
- 2 scoops calcium and magnesium powder (Skin Friend PM, optional)

Heat the milk in a saucepan along with the saffron strands and simmer on low for 5 minutes. Add the calcium/magnesium if using. Allow to stand for up to 5 minutes to infuse the saffron, then serve warm. Eat the saffron strands for the full benefits.

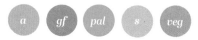

Healthy Skin Juice

Serves 2, preparation time 5 minutes

The secret to a healthy skin juice is more vegies and a special combination of gut-soothing fruit. This highly alkalizing drink is designed to reduce inflammation, promote acid–alkaline balance in your body and aid liver detoxification.

- 1 large stalk celery
- 3 large carrots, tops removed (S)
- ½ beetroot/beet (peeled) (S)
- 1 ripe pear
- ½ cup fresh papaya, chopped (skin and seeds discarded) (A)

Wash, scrub and chop up the vegetables and fruit. Using a juicing machine, juice the ingredients, ending by adding a splash of filtered or spring water.

If you are using a cold-pressed juicing machine or a 'slow juicer', pour the juice through the juicer again to remove more of the pulp (or strain it) or drink it with the pulp as it is good for you.

Serve immediately or use within 6 hours.

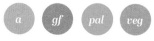

Papaya Flaxseed Drink: dry skin remedy

1 day's supply for one adult, preparation time 3 minutes (overnight freezing time is optional)

Papaya Flaxseed Drink contains omega-3 rich flaxseed oil with a twist ... It is teamed with lecithin, which acts like an oil emulsifier to make it easier for your body to utilize the omega-3 oils. If you are sensitive to amines, you could use peeled frozen pear pieces instead of papaya. This is a low salicylate drink. Add Skin Friend AM if you have skin inflammation or acne.

- 1½ cups chilled filtered or spring water
- 1 cup chopped papaya, skin and seeds discarded (pre-freeze for a cold drink) (A)
- 1 teaspoon sunflower lecithin granules (non-GMO, optional)
- ½–1 teaspoon organic flaxseed oil (begin on low dose) 2 ice cubes

Combine all the ingredients in a high-speed blender and blend until smooth.

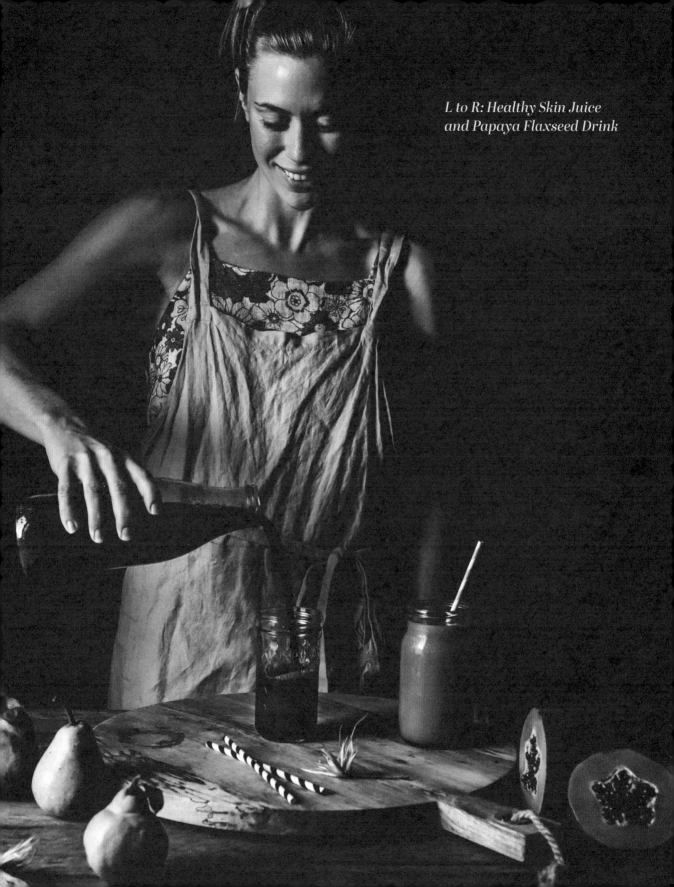

L to R: Healthy Skin Juice
and Papaya Flaxseed Drink

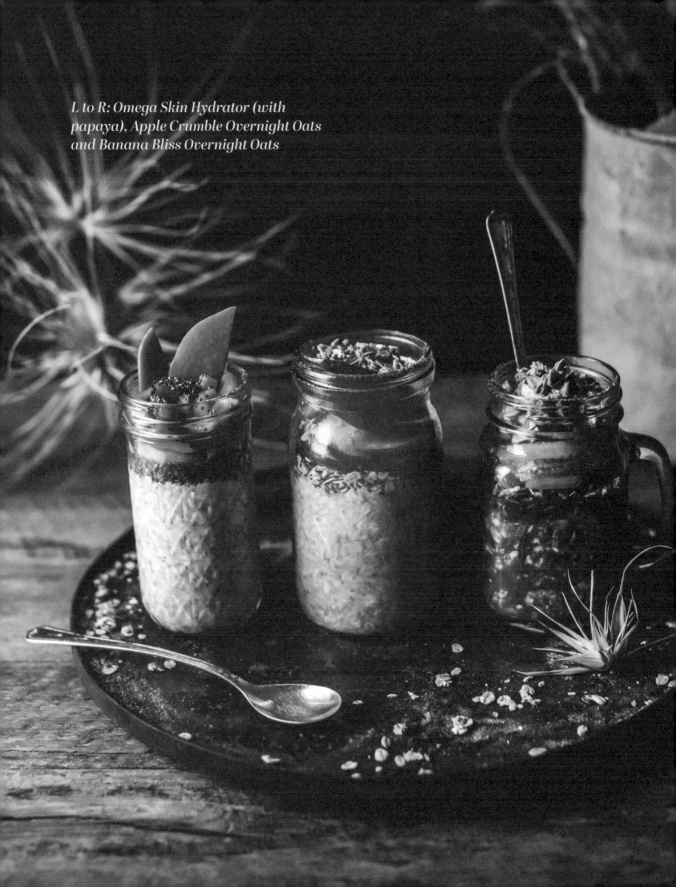

L to R: Omega Skin Hydrator (with papaya), Apple Crumble Overnight Oats and Banana Bliss Overnight Oats

Chapter 11
Breakfast and snacks

Overnight Oats

Serves 2, preparation time 3 minutes

This simple recipe is a household favourite and I consumed Overnight Oats (without fruit) during my recovery from eczema. Prepare two jars at a time and keep them in the refrigerator for two breakfasts or handy snacks. You don't need to eat a whole serve all at once: you can put the leftovers back into the refrigerator and save them for dessert, as oats promote satiety and a better night's sleep. See Variations.

- 2 cups rolled oats (ideally organic; gluten-free only if necessary)
- 2 cups organic oat milk
- *Optional low salicylate topping:* ½ ripe pear, peeled, core removed and sliced

You will need two jars or breakfast bowls. Place 1 cup of oats into each jar/bowl and then pour 1 cup of milk into each jar. Cover with reusable silicon covers, plastic wrap or lids and place into the refrigerator overnight. At breakfast, add extra milk and top it with sliced peeled pear (this is the low salicylate topping option). Use the second jar within 2–3 days and add the topping just before serving.

Variation 1: Omega Skin Hydrator

Serves 1, preparation time 3 minutes

Place into a jar or bowl 1 cup of rolled oats, 1 cup of oat milk (or see 'Milk options for your skin type', p. 92), and 1 teaspoon of whole (or ground) flaxseeds, chia seeds or hemp seeds. Cover and soak overnight. Before serving, add more milk and top with sliced banana or papaya (and 1 teaspoon of maple syrup, if desired).

Variation 2: Apple Crumble Overnight Oats

Serves 1, preparation time 3 minutes

Place into a jar or bowl 1 cup of rolled oats, 1 cup of oat milk (or see 'Milk options for your skin type', p. 92), cover and soak overnight. Before serving, add more milk and top with Golden Granola (p. 129) and finely sliced Red Delicious apple (mix in 1 teaspoon of maple syrup, if desired).

Variation 3: Banana Bliss Overnight Oats

Serves 1, preparation time 3 minutes

Place into a jar 1 tablespoon of carob powder, 1 teaspoon of maple syrup and 1–2 tablespoons of boiling hot water and mix until smooth. Then add 1 cup of rolled oats, 1 cup of oat milk (or see 'Milk options for your skin type', p. 92), mix, cover and soak overnight. Before serving, add more milk and top it with maple fried banana (sliced banana pan fried in a little maple syrup or simply use raw fresh banana slices.

Papaya Sunrise Porridge

Serves 1 adult, preparation time 3 minutes, cooking time 5 minutes (soaking overnight is optional)

Soothe your skin and digestive tract and make your heart happy with the goodness of oats and papaya. Note that hemp seeds and chia seeds contain salicylates and amines, so they are optional. See Variation (below) for a gluten-free quinoa porridge recipe. Toppings: pear is the low amine/histamine option and all the mentioned fruits are low in salicylates. If you are following Menu 4, omit the seeds and use peeled pear instead of papaya.

- ¾ cup rolled oats
- 1 teaspoon hemp seeds or chia seeds (optional) (S) (A)
- ½ cup organic oat milk or filtered or spring water, or plant-based milk of choice (p. 92)
- ½ cup sliced papaya, skin and seeds removed (A), or ½ pear, peeled and sliced

Optional overnight soaking to increase the goodness: place the oats and seeds into a bowl and cover with about 1 cup of water. Cover the bowl with plastic wrap or a silicon cover and place it in the refrigerator overnight.

In the morning, pour the oats into a small saucepan, add the milk and heat until it thickens, stirring often. Add more milk as needed. Serve with extra milk and top with sliced papaya. I don't add any sweetener but feel free to drizzle ½–1 teaspoon of maple syrup if desired.

Variation: Quinoa Porridge

Rinse ½ cup white quinoa (not puffed), and simmer on low in 1 cup of water or plant-based milk of choice until thick (about 12–15 minutes). Add 1 teaspoon of maple syrup and serve with sliced papaya, pawpaw, pear or banana.

*Papaya Sunrise Porridge
with chia seeds, oat milk and
Carob Nutella (p. 141)*

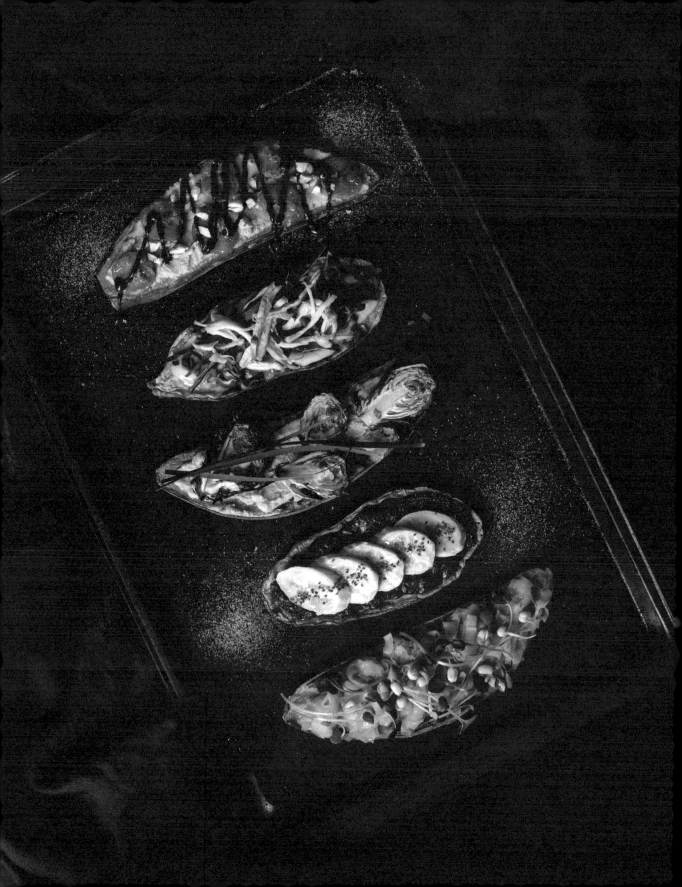

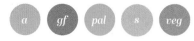

Sweet Potato Toast

Serves 2, preparation time 10 minutes, cooking time 7–10 minutes

I love roasted sweet potato and this recipe uses the humble toaster so it takes less than 10 minutes to cook (although you have the option to roast the sweet potato slices with a little oil, which will take about 30 minutes).

1 large, wide sweet potato, ends trimmed (choose a good shape for slicing) (S)

Savoury toppings to choose from:

- Cashew Butter (p. 141) (H)
- Sesame-free Hummus (p. 145) and grated fresh beetroot/beets (S) (H)
- Caramelized Leek Sauce (p. 142) and mung bean sprouts or pea sprouts
- Cashew Butter (p. 141)with cooked skinless chicken and red cabbage (H)

Sweet toppings to choose from:

- Sliced fried banana (A) with Salted Caramel Nut Butter (p. 141) (H)
- Fresh banana (A) and Carob Nutella (p. 141) (H)
- Roasted Maple Brussel Bites, sliced (p. 132)

Wash and scrub the sweet potato (peel if necessary), and slice it lengthwise into even slices, just under 1 cm (½ in) thick. You should have 3–4 slices.

Adjust your toaster setting to high. Place the slices into the toaster and toast them several times until they reach the desired softness. When you remove them remember to reduce your toaster setting back to the original setting to ensure you don't burn regular toast in the future.

Spread with nut butter or hummus and then top them with your toppings of choice.

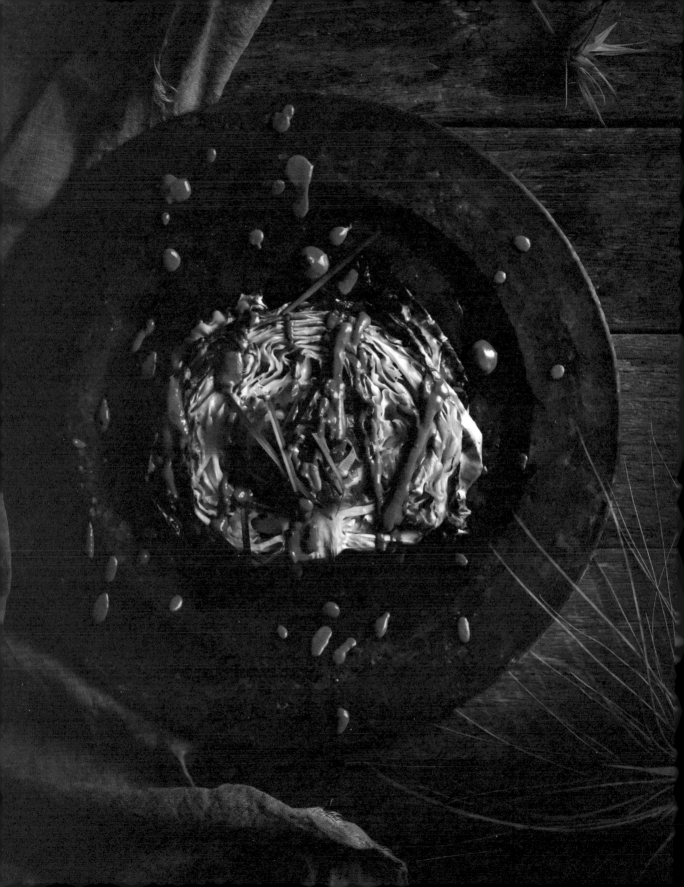

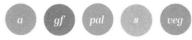

Cabbage Steaks with Beet Cream

Makes 5–6 steaks, combined preparation and cooking time 45 minutes

Who knew cabbage could taste this good? When roasted, cabbage becomes a flavourful 'steak' that is both soft and crunchy. Topped with caramelized leeks and a creamy beetroot sauce, this makes a healthy and delicious breakfast, lunch or side dish with dinner. If you are allergic to cashews, replace the Beet Cream with White Bean Sauce (p. 146) and add some fresh grated beetroot during the mixing process. Note that beets contain moderate salicylates so leave out this ingredient if you need to, and use red cabbage instead of white to get a splash of low-sal colour.

- 1 small–medium whole white cabbage
- ½ serve Beet Cream (p. 163) (S) (H)
- 2 teaspoons oil (see 'Cooking oil options for your skin type', p. 92)
- 1 teaspoon garlic powder
- ½ serve Caramelized Leek Sauce (p. 142)
- handful of green spring onions (shallots, scallions) or chives

Preheat a fan-forced oven to 180°C (350°F) and line a baking tray with a silicon mat or baking (parchment) paper and set aside.
If making the Beet Cream, soak the cashews in boiling hot water now.

Using a knife, remove the outer green layers of the cabbage and trim the stem/base so the cabbage can stand up flat on the bench. Cut 1.5 cm (½ in) thick slices so you have about 5 or 6 'steaks'. Rinse them in water so they are damp, then using a pastry brush (or your fingers), brush the oil onto both sides of the steaks. Place them onto the tray and sprinkle one side with the garlic powder. Bake the cabbage in the oven for about 20 minutes, then carefully turn them over and bake for another 20 minutes. Check them every 5 minutes to ensure they don't burn.

Meanwhile, finish making the Beet Cream and the Caramelized Leek Sauce.

The cabbage is ready when it is soft in the middle and easy to pierce with a knife. Place the steaks onto plates and top them with the Caramelized Leek Sauce and spring onions or chives, then drizzle with Beet Cream. Store the leftovers in a sealed container in the refrigerator (and reheat them when needed).

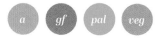

Papaya Beauty Smoothie Bowl

Serves 1, preparation time 5 minutes (pre-freeze papaya overnight)

This beauty smoothie bowl has a sublime flavour and a smooth consistency that reminds me of whipped mango mousse. Note the cashews must be soaked overnight in water to enable a smooth consistency. Double this recipe to make two batches for consecutive breakfasts. If you can't eat cashews, use ½ cup frozen banana instead.

- ½ cup soaked raw cashews (H)
- 1 cup papaya, skin and seeds removed, sliced and pre-frozen (A)
- 1 cup cashew milk (H) or plant-based milk of choice (p. 92)
- 2 scoops Skin Friend AM (optional)
- 1 teaspoon rice syrup or real maple syrup

Optional toppings:
- 1 teaspoon chia seeds, hemp seeds or flaxseeds/linseeds (S) (A)
- eczema-friendly fruits: sliced banana (A) papaya (A) or peeled pear
- Golden Granola (p. 129)

Soak the cashews in water in a sealed container to soften and activate them overnight (or freeze banana), and freeze the diced papaya. The next day, place the papaya, soaked cashews, milk optional multivitamin and rice or maple syrup into a high-speed blender and blend on high until smooth. Pour into a bowl and either allow time for it to set by placing it into the freezer for 10–15 minutes, or consume immediately.

When ready to serve, top the smoothie bowl with seeds and fruit of choice or Golden Granola.

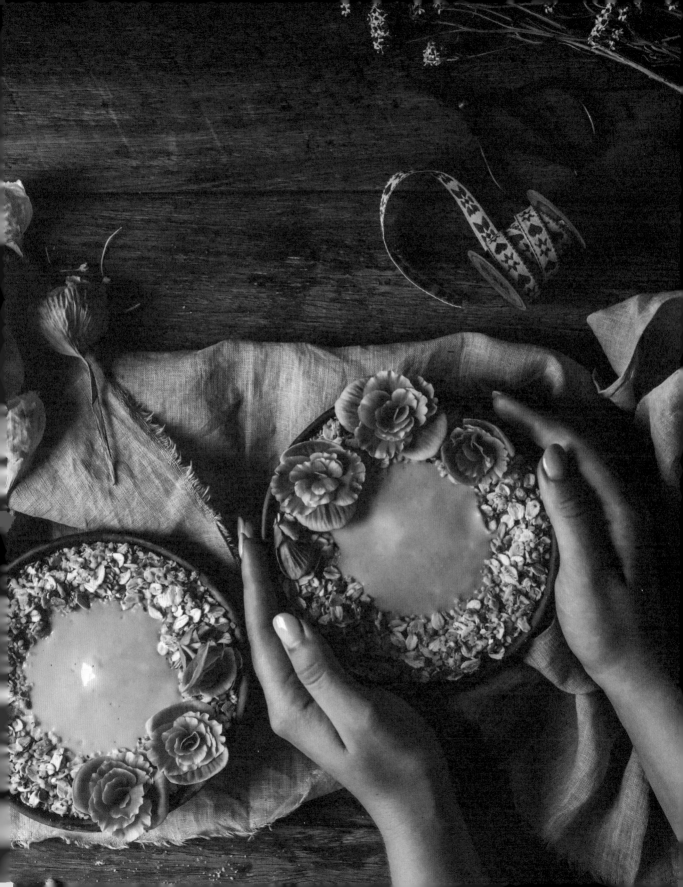

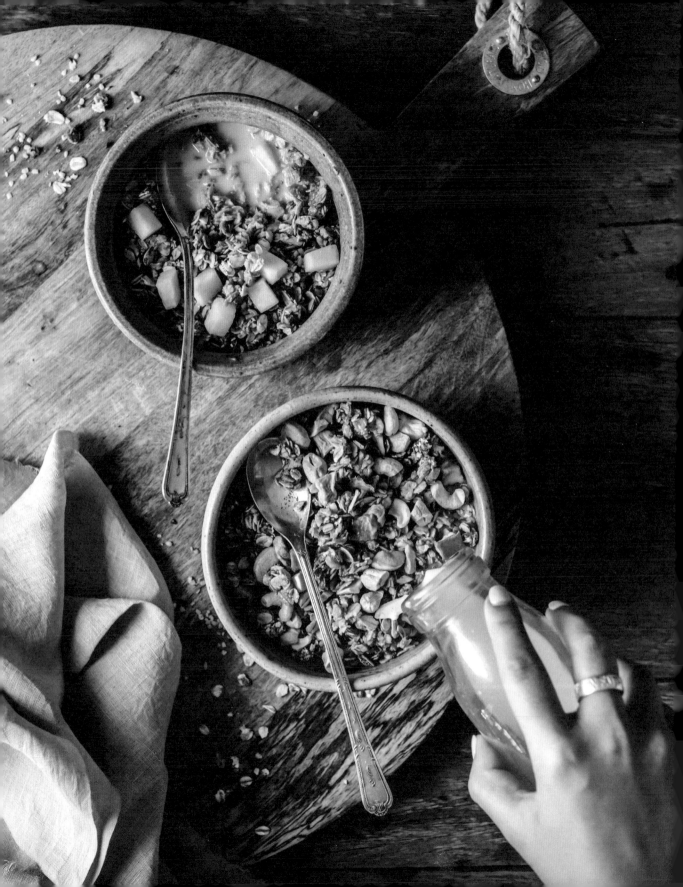

Golden Granola

Makes 4 servings, preparation time 15 minutes, cooking time 20 minutes

Make your own healthy granola with this simple recipe. If you are following Menu 4 you can have the granola with peeled fresh pear (avoid the optional extras). If you have eczema, skin rashes or amine sensitivity, omit the cashews.

- 4 cups organic rolled oats (G)
- 2 cups quinoa flakes
- 4 tablespoons rice malt syrup (brown rice syrup)

Optional extras:
- 4 tablespoons chia seeds, flaxseeds (linseeds) or hemp seeds
- ½ cup sliced dried pear or apple (SS) (check the dried fruits are preservative-free)
- 1 cup raw cashews, crushed (H)

Preheat the oven to 180°C (350°F) and line a large baking tray with a silicon mat or baking (parchment) paper and set aside.

Using a medium-sized bowl, mix the oats and quinoa flakes.

Heat the rice syrup in a small saucepan on medium heat until the syrup becomes runny, then drizzle the syrup onto the oat mix and stir until combined. Pour the mixture onto the tray and spread it out evenly. Place the tray into the oven and cook the mixture for 20 minutes or until slightly golden (do not overcook).

Remove the tray from the oven and allow the mixture to cool. Then place it into a container and mix in the optional ingredients. Seal tightly with a lid and use within a month. Serve with plant-based milk of choice (p. 92) and fresh peeled pear.

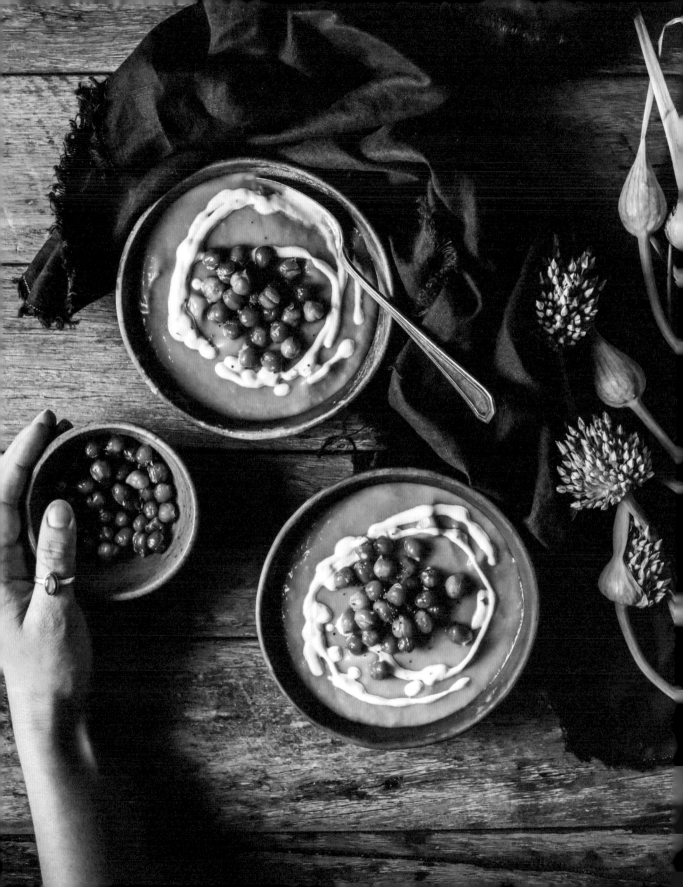

Roasted Chickpeas

Makes 4 servings, preparation time 5 minutes, cooking time 30 minutes

Roasted chickpeas (garbanzo beans) and roasted black beans (see Variation, below) are a low GI, protein-rich snack that is easy to make. Pop them into your lunchbox or sprinkle them onto salads such as Cashew Caesar Salad (p. 170), Quinoa Nourish Bowl (p. 166) and soups such as Green Detox Soup (p. 179) and Beet Detox Soup (p. 149).

- 1 x 400 g (14 oz) can organic chickpeas (garbanzo beans) drained and rinsed
- 1 teaspoon oil (refer to 'Cooking oil options for your skin type', p. 92)
- ¼ teaspoon quality sea salt (fine, not coarse)

Preheat the oven to 200°C (400°F) and line a large baking tray with a silicon mat or baking (parchment) paper and set aside.

Drain and rinse the chickpeas thoroughly in fresh water using a strainer/colander and gently pat dry with a clean tea towel. Place the chickpeas into a sealable container along with the oil and salt, secure the lid and gently shake to evenly coat the chickpeas with the seasoning and oil. Then spread the chickpeas in a single layer on the tray. Bake for 20 minutes, then roughly attempt to flip over the chickpeas with an egg flip and cook for another 10 minutes or until crunchy. Serve warm or cold and store the remainder in a sealed container in the refrigerator.

Variation: Roasted Black Beans

Combine 1 can of organic black beans, which have been drained, rinsed and dried with a clean tea towel, with 1 teaspoon of oil (refer to 'Cooking oil options for your skin type', p. 92) and ¼ teaspoon quality sea salt (fine, not coarse). Refer to the Roasted Chickpeas instructions above and bake for 30 minutes or until crispy.

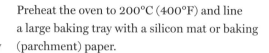

Roasted Maple Brussel Bites

Serves 4 as a snack, preparation time 7 minutes, cooking time 20 minutes

Hello, new love of my life. I hated Brussels sprouts until I learnt how to roast them like this. I often make this recipe without the maple syrup for a savoury dish. Serve them on their own or with White Bean Sauce (p. 146) and Lamb Skewers (p. 164) or Crispy Chicken (p. 184).

- 10 medium Brussels sprouts, stalk end trimmed
- 1 tablespoon rice bran oil or sunflower oil (low salicylate oils; or refer to 'Cooking oil options for your skin type', p. 92)
- 1 tablespoon real maple syrup
- ¼ teaspoon quality sea salt

Preheat the oven to 200°C (400°F) and line a large baking tray with a silicon mat or baking (parchment) paper.

Wash the Brussels sprouts and slice them in half lengthwise, then place them into a dry saucepan or container with a lid, drizzle on the oil, maple syrup and salt. Cover with a lid then shake the pot to evenly coat the sprouts.

Spread the Brussels sprouts onto the tray and bake them in the oven for 20 minutes or until softened and lightly browned, turning them over after 10 minutes using tongs. Serve them warm or hot.

Make your own mini Brussel Burgers by fashioning organic beef mince into mini burger patties (just add a sprinkle of salt); then cook and secure them with a toothpick between cooked Brussels sprouts and serve them warm.

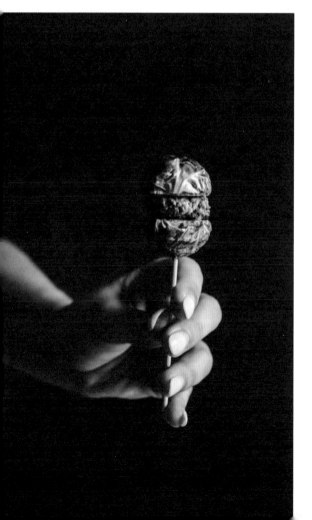

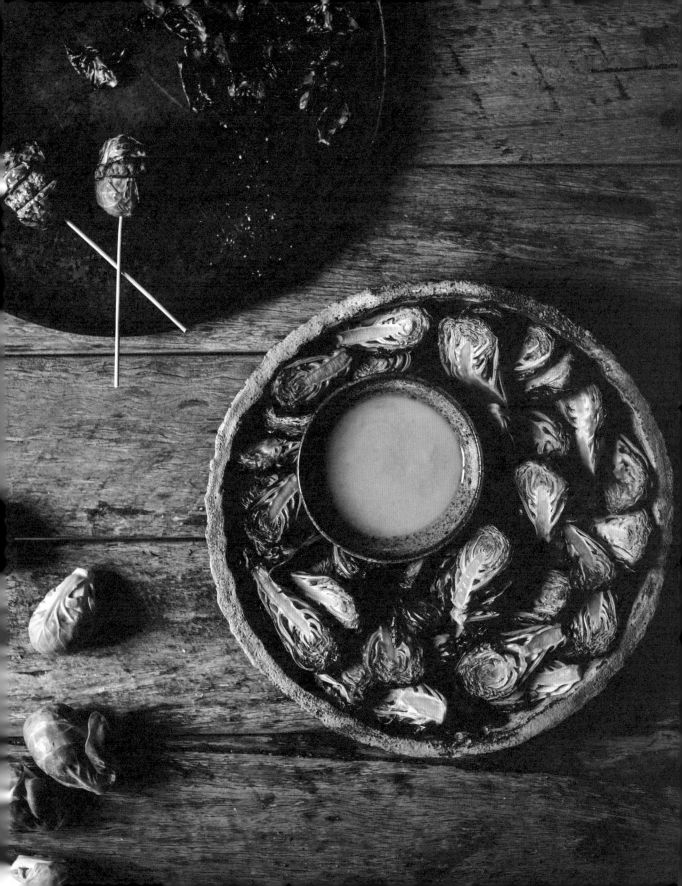

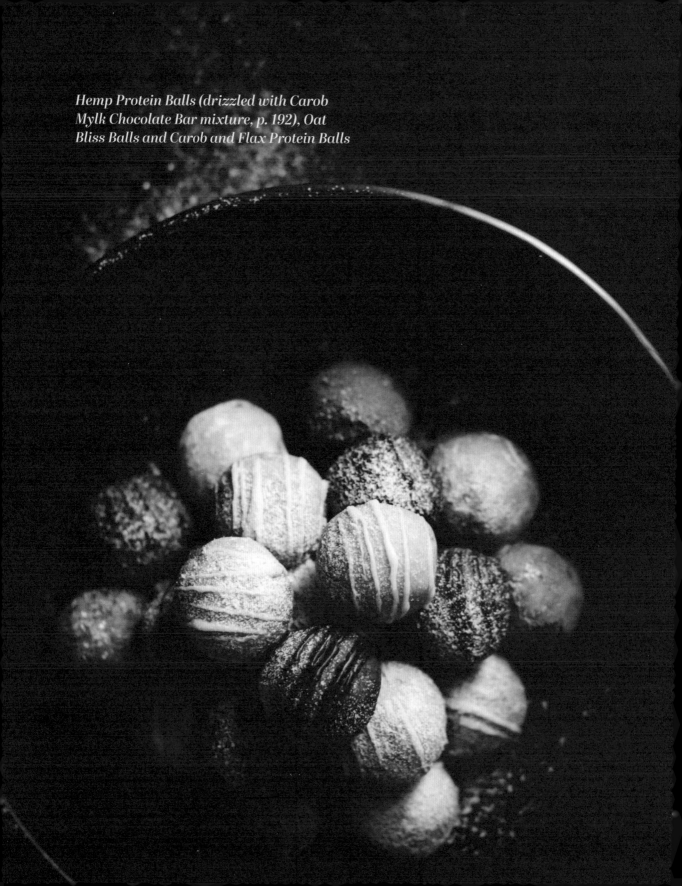

Hemp Protein Balls (drizzled with Carob
Mylk Chocolate Bar mixture, p. 192), Oat
Bliss Balls and Carob and Flax Protein Balls

Hemp Protein Balls

Makes 16 balls, preparation time 30 minutes, setting time 2 hours

Hello strong nails, better bones and healthy hair. This high-protein recipe is my go-to for strengthening my nails and hair — you will see and feel the difference. I have also made this recipe using oat flour, instead of pea protein powder (note that oats usually contain gluten). See optional toppings on p. 136.

- ¼ cup cacao butter
- 1 cup pea protein powder (or oat flour — contains gluten)
- ½ cup rice protein powder (or oat flour — contains gluten)
- ½ cup hemp protein powder (A)
- 2–3 tablespoons pure maple syrup or rice malt/brown rice syrup (optional)
- ⅓ cup plant-based milk of choice (p. 92)

Line a large flat container that has a lid (approximately 20 x 25 cm/8 x 10 in) with baking (parchment) paper and set aside. Alternatively, you can use two smaller containers.

Melt the cacao butter on medium heat, using the double-boil method described on p. 192. If you are using rice malt syrup, melt it with the cacao butter. When melted, remove the bowl from the heat and allow it to slightly cool.

Place the remaining ingredients into a food processor, then pour in the cacao butter and process briefly. Scrape down the sides with a spatula or a butter knife, place the lid back on and process again, (ideally) until a dough ball forms. Stop processing immediately when a large dough ball appears. The dough should easily press into balls and not stick to your hands or the side of the machine. If the dough is too sticky add a little more flour or protein powder; if it forms lots of tiny dough balls it is too dry so add 1 tablespoon of plant-based milk at a time and mix again, until one dough ball forms or until smooth.

Using clean hands and a tablespoon, scoop 1 tablespoon of the mixture and roll it into a ball, and repeat the process. Place the balls into the container. Place the lid on the container and store it in the refrigerator. The balls take 2 hours to set but if you are keen to try them now, place a couple into the freezer for 10 minutes.

Variation: Oat Bliss Balls

Makes 20 balls, preparation time 30 minutes, setting time 2 hours

Melt ¼ cup of cacao butter using the double-boil method described on p. 192. Then in a food processor place 2½ cups of oat flour, 3 tablespoons maple syrup (or less — here's the variation for Menu 4: 2 tablespoons maple syrup and 1 tablespoon oat milk), ½ cup oat milk and the melted cacao butter and blend until a dough ball forms. Refer to Hemp Protein Balls recipe above for further instructions.

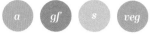

Carob and Flax Protein Balls

Makes 20–22 balls, preparation time 30 minutes, setting time 2 hours

This is a fabulous protein-rich recipe for creating strong nails, better bones and healthy hair. See optional toppings below.

- ⅓ cup cacao butter
- 1 cup raw cashews, unsalted (H)
- ¼ cup real maple syrup
- 1 cup pea protein powder (or ½ cup pea protein powder and ½ cup rice protein powder)
- ⅓ cup roasted carob powder
- 1 tablespoon whole flaxseeds/linseeds (S) (A)
- pinch of quality sea salt (optional)

Using the double-boil method described on p. 192, melt the cacao butter then remove from the heat to slightly cool.

Process the raw cashews in a food processor and blend until they become a fine meal or nut butter. To help this process you can gradually add the maple syrup and blend until smooth. Stop the motor and scrape down the sides with a spatula or butter knife. Then add the protein powder/s, carob powder, melted cacao butter, flaxseeds and salt (if using) and briefly mix in the food processor. Scrape the sides and blend again. The mixture should form a large ball while blending — if tiny balls form, the mixture is too dry. If it is a little too dry, add a tablespoon at a time of plant-based milk (see p. 92 for options) and mix briefly. If the mixture is too wet it will stick to the sides — if this occurs, let it sit for 5 minutes and see if it firms up.

Line a large flat container with baking (parchment) paper (to prevent sticking). Using clean hands and a tablespoon, scoop 1 tablespoon of the mixture and roll it into a ball, place onto the paper and repeat the process. Cover the container with a lid and store it in the refrigerator. The balls will take about 2 hours to set but if you are keen to try them now, place a couple into the freezer for 10 minutes.

Optional toppings: I like these plain but optional toppings include crushed raw cashews or a drizzle of Carob Mylk Chocolate (p. 192).

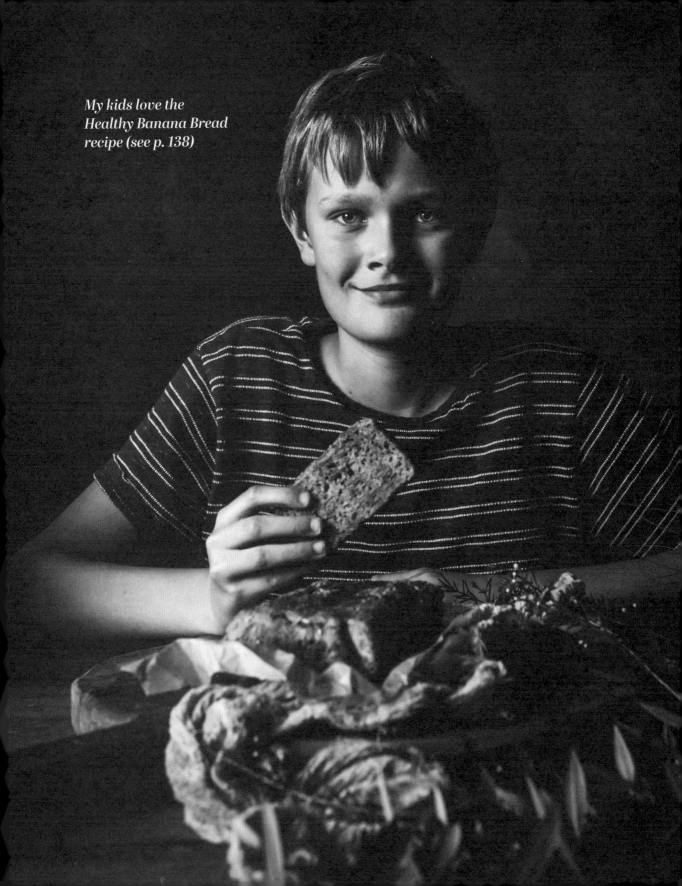

My kids love the Healthy Banana Bread recipe (see p. 138)

Healthy Banana Bread

Makes 1 loaf, preparation time 20 minutes, cooking time 50 minutes

Healthy cake? There is such a thing ... it's called Healthy Banana Bread, which is like a dense cake packed with fibre-filled, potassium-rich bananas and the goodness of wholemeal spelt. Feel free to swap the spelt flour with gluten-free all-purpose flour if you are gluten intolerant. This clever recipe is egg- and dairy-free: the arrowroot flour binds it all together nicely. Serve me for breakfast or dessert topped with Cashew Butter (p. 141, but it's even good on its own). Tip: use bananas that are ripe enough for mashing and choose regular bananas, not Lady Finger/sugar bananas as they are rich in salicylates.

- 1 cup wholemeal/wholewheat spelt flour (or gluten-free plain/all-purpose flour)
- ½ cup arrowroot starch/flour (or tapioca starch)
- 3 teaspoons baking powder
- 3 ripe bananas, mashed (A)
- ½ cup real maple syrup (plus extra to drizzle)
- 1 tablespoon rice bran oil or see p. 92 for best oils for your skin type
- 1–2 teaspoons chia seeds (optional: S, A)

Preheat the oven to 180°C (350°F) or a fan forced oven to 170°C (325°F) and line a rectangular loaf tin (approx. 13 x 24 cm/5 x 9½ in) with baking (parchment) paper.

In a medium bowl, combine the two flours and baking powder and mix well (you can sift the flour mix if desired). In a separate flat-based bowl, mash the bananas with a potato masher or a fork, then stir in the maple syrup and oil and mix. Add the wet ingredients to the dry ingredients and fold together — don't overmix.

Pour the mixture into the lined tin and spread the batter evenly. Then sprinkle on the chia seeds, if using. Bake for 40–50 minutes or until set and golden on top. It may seem a little undercooked when it comes out but it will continue cooking once out so don't overcook it.

When serving, cut thick slices (about 2 cm/1 in thick) and toast in a toaster or lightly fry in a pan until golden on each side. Or simply pop a slice into your lunchbox and serve it cold. Optional: top with Cashew Butter (p. 141).

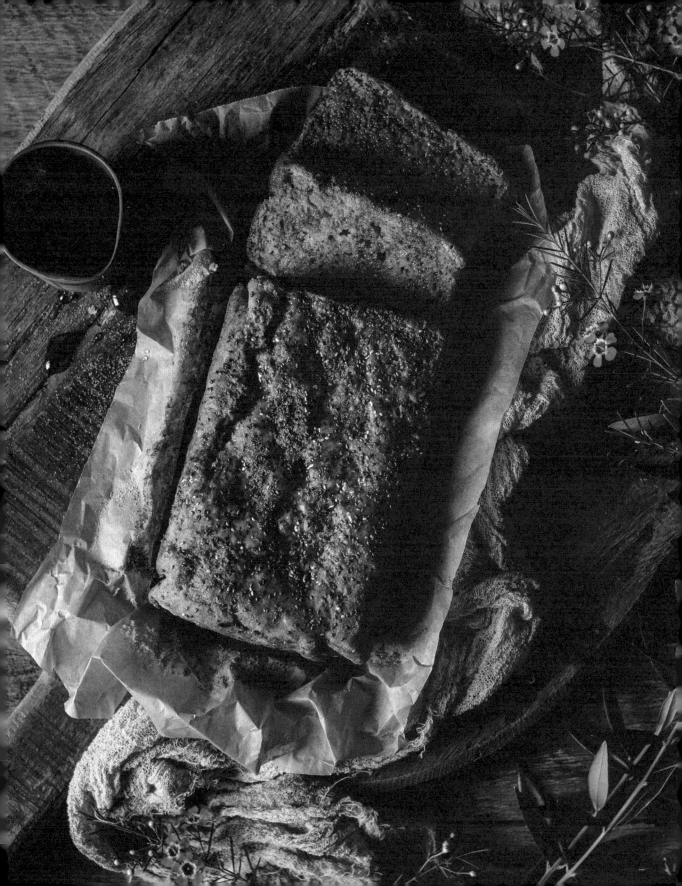

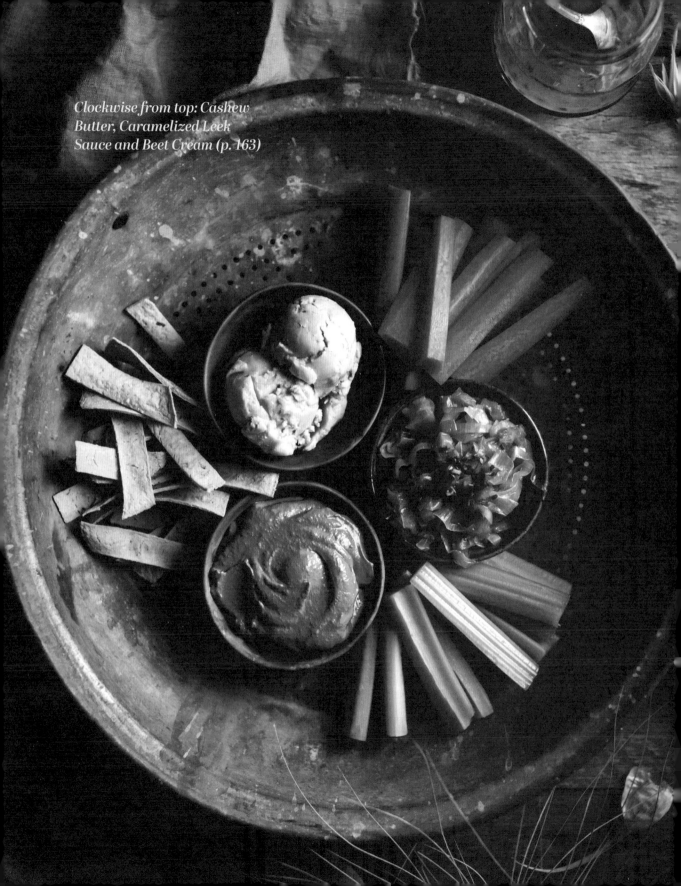

Clockwise from top: Cashew Butter, Caramelized Leek Sauce and Beet Cream (p. 163)

Chapter 12
Sauces, spreads and dips

Cashew Butter

Makes 1 jar, preparation time 10 minutes

This delicious nutty spread is a fantastic butter and margarine substitute and (in my humble opinion) it's much nicer than almond butter. Spread this mineral-rich butter onto celery sticks or toast, such as Sweet Potato Toast (p. 123).

- 1½ cups raw cashews (unsalted, do not soak) (H)
- 2 teaspoons oil (refer to 'Cooking oil options for your skin type', p. 92)
- ¼ teaspoon quality sea salt

Place the cashews, oil and salt into a high-speed food processor or nut butter blender and blend on high until it resembles breadcrumbs. Be patient as it can take time for the spread to liquefy. Frequently switch off the food processor and scrape down the sides then blend again until it forms a thick spread. If it turns into a ball, continue to blend it and then scrape down the sides.

Once the spread has thinned out and is fairly smooth, transfer it to a clean/dry jar or container, seal with a lid and store in the refrigerator.

Cashew Butter can be kept for 2–3 weeks in the refrigerator, or maybe longer if you have sterilized the jar and lid correctly. It probably won't last that long … I eat mine pretty quickly.

Variation: Salted Caramel Nut Butter

Make Cashew Butter as above and add 3 teaspoons of real maple syrup, 2 tablespoons of filtered or spring water, ½ teaspoon of carob powder and two pinches of coarse sea salt (optional) during the processing stage for a sweet and salty nut butter which is perfect for spreading onto toast or piped onto Banana Popsicles (p. 191). Use within 10 days.

Variation: Carob Nutella

In a food processor, make Cashew Butter as above, then add 2 tablespoons of maple syrup, 2 tablespoons of carob powder, a pinch of quality sea salt and 2–3 tablespoons of plant-based milk (see p. 92 for milk options) and process until smooth. Store in a jar in the refrigerator for up to 10 days.

Cashew Cream

Makes 1 batch, preparation time 15 minutes (plus soaking time)

A drizzle of Cashew Cream makes savoury dishes look good and taste great — that's why it features in so many of my food photos. Use a squeezie sauce bottle to get the perfect drizzle every time.

- 1 cup raw cashews, unsalted (H)
- ¾ cup filtered or spring water
- ¼ teaspoon quality sea salt
- ¼ teaspoon garlic powder (optional)

Activation soaking method: if you have time, soak the cashews overnight in warm water to activate the cashews — ideally do not soak them for more than 6 hours. Quick soaking method:

pour boiling water onto the cashews and soak them for about 30 minutes or until they are soft and swollen.

After soaking, drain and rinse the cashews well using fresh water. Place them into a high-speed blender along with the water, salt and garlic powder, if using, and blend on high until smooth. Store in an airtight jar or squeezie sauce bottle in the refrigerator for up to 4 days.

Variation: Beet Cream

Make Cashew Cream as above, and during the blending process add 2–3 tablespoons of grated fresh beetroot, until the desired colour is reached.

Caramelized Leek Sauce

Makes 1 cup, preparation time 3 minutes, cooking time 7 minutes

This chunky and deliciously sweet sauce makes any dish taste amazing. It is a perfect accompaniment for lamb or beef, San Choy Bau (p. 159), fish, Soft Tacos (p. 153) and potato dishes, or make your own stir-fry topped with this flavoursome sauce.

- 1 medium leek, green leafy part removed, end trimmed
- 1 tablespoon filtered or spring water
- 1–2 tablespoons real maple syrup
- ⅛ teaspoon quality sea salt

Wash the leek layers to remove the dirt then finely slice the white parts and palest green parts of the leek. Heat the water in a saucepan on medium heat, and sauté the leek until very soft. Add the maple syrup and sea salt and cook on low heat for another few minutes until it's sticky and golden.

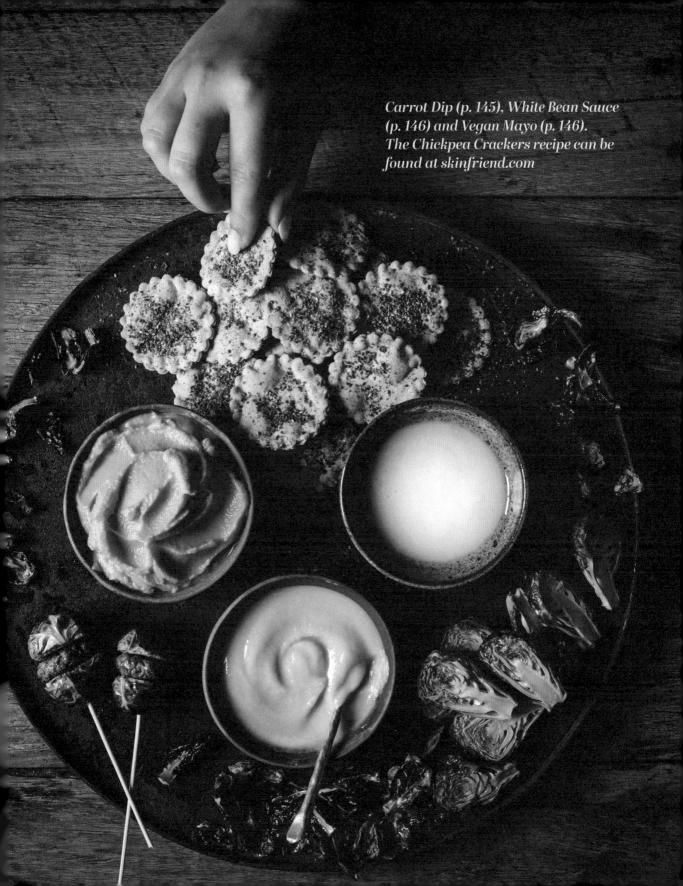

Carrot Dip (p. 145), White Bean Sauce (p. 146) and Vegan Mayo (p. 146). The Chickpea Crackers recipe can be found at *skinfriend.com*

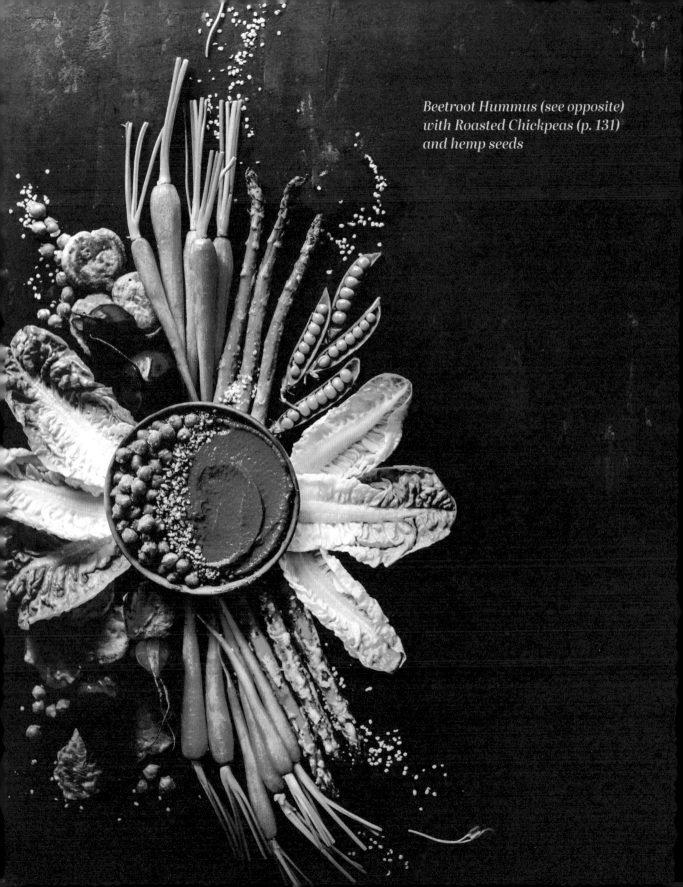

Beetroot Hummus (see opposite)
with Roasted Chickpeas (p. 131)
and hemp seeds

Sesame-free Hummus

Makes 1 cup, preparation time 10 minutes

Chickpeas (garbanzo beans) make a lovely protein-rich dip that can be used to accompany crackers and vegie sticks. Use a dollop on salads or spread it onto Sweet Potato Toast (p. 123) for a healthy snack, breakfast or lunch.

- 1 x 400 g (14 oz) can organic chickpeas (garbanzo beans), drained and rinsed
- 1 small clove garlic, minced (begin with ½ and adjust to taste)
- 1 tablespoon rice bran oil (or refer to 'Cooking oil options for your skin type', p. 92)
- 5 tablespoons (100 ml/3–4 fl oz) filtered or spring water
- ⅛ teaspoon quality sea salt (canned chickpeas are salty so adjust to taste)

Place all the ingredients into a food processor and blend until smooth. Store the dip in a sealed container in the refrigerator. Hummus will last for 4–5 days.

Variation: Beetroot Hummus

Make Sesame-free Hummus as above. Then peel and grate a small fresh beetroot (S) and add 2–3 tablespoons of the grated beetroot to the hummus and blend until smooth.

Carrot Dip

Makes 1½ cups, preparation time 5 minutes, cooking time 15 minutes

Carrots are a rich source of skin-loving beta-carotene, which converts to vitamin A and helps to protect your skin from sun damage and dehydration. This lovely dip can be served with plain rice crackers and celery sticks.

- 2 large carrots, peeled (S)
- ½ cup canned chickpeas (garbanzo beans)
- ¼ teaspoon garlic powder (or ¼ clove fresh garlic, minced)
- 2 teaspoons oil (refer to 'Cooking oil options for your skin type', p. 92)
- ¼ teaspoon quality sea salt
- 3 tablespoons filtered or spring water

Chop the carrots — you will need one heaped cup for the recipe — and place them into a steamer and cook until they are very soft (about 15 minutes). Drain and allow them to partially cool.

Meanwhile, drain and rinse the chickpeas then place them with the remaining ingredients into a high-speed blender and blend on high until smooth. Add 1–2 tablespoons of extra water for a thinner consistency if necessary, and mix. Store in a sealed container in the refrigerator for up to 4 days.

White Bean Sauce

Makes 1 cup, preparation time 10 minutes, cooking time 5 minutes

White Bean Sauce is a tasty, protein-rich alternative to Cashew Cream. It makes a great companion to savoury recipes including Lamb Skewers (p. 164), Quinoa Nourish Bowl (p. 166), Sweet Potato Nourish Bowl (p. 169), Cashew Caesar Salad (p. 170) and Crispy Sweet Potato Gnocchi (p. 174).

- 1 cup canned white beans
- ½ cup filtered or spring water
- ½ teaspoon quality sea salt
- ¼ teaspoon of ascorbic acid or citric acid (for tang, optional)
- ½ small clove fresh garlic, peeled and minced (or ½ teaspoon dried garlic powder)

Drain and rinse the beans with plenty of water and shake off the excess water. Place the beans, water, salt and other ingredients into a high-speed blender and blend on high until smooth. Use a squeezie sauce bottle to drizzle the sauce onto meals. Store in an airtight container in the refrigerator for up to 3 days.

Vegan Mayo

Makes 1 serving, preparation time 5 minutes

Vegan Mayo is about to change your life. This rich, creamy mayo is ready in only 5 minutes and it tastes great. You will need ½ cup of aquafaba, which is the drained water (brine) from a can of chickpeas/garbanzo beans (so don't make home-cooked chickpeas for this recipe). The leftover chickpeas can be used to make Sesame-free Hummus (p. 145) or Roasted Chickpeas (p. 131) for a tasty snack or salad topping. Serve Vegan Mayo with savoury dishes such as Asparagus and Black Bean Soft Tacos (p. 155), Crispy Chicken (p. 184), Cabbage Steaks (p. 125), Quinoa Nourish Bowl (p. 166).

- ½ cup aquafaba from 1 x 400g (14 oz) can of chickpeas (garbanzo beans)
- 1 cup raw cashews, unsoaked (H)
- ½ teaspoon of citric acid or ascorbic acid
- ½ teaspoon quality sea salt
- ½ teaspoon garlic powder or 1 clove garlic
- 5 teaspoons oil (refer to 'Cooking oil options for your skin type', p. 92)

Open the can of chickpeas and, using a strainer, drain the chickpea water into a bowl. Measure ½ cup of this water (aquafaba/brine) and pour it into a high-speed blender, or use a stick blender, and blend on high for about 1 minute to create a frothy mixture. Add the remaining ingredients and blend on high until the mixture is smooth and creamy. Store in the refrigerator in a sealed container or sterilized jar. Vegan Mayo will last for up to 5 days if refrigerated.

Omega Salad Dressing

Makes 1 cup, preparation time 5 minutes

This sweet and savoury dressing contains beauty-boosting omega-3 from flaxseed oil and alkalizing apple cider vinegar (ACV), which contains antibacterial and antifungal compounds — ACV is fermented and not suitable for people with sulphite sensitivity or histamine/salicylate intolerance. Drizzle this dressing on salads or Quinoa Nourish Bowl (p. 166). For an amine-free and salicylate-free dressing, see Variation, below.

- ⅓ cup extra virgin olive oil (SS, AA; or refer to 'Cooking oil options for your skin type', p. 92)
- ⅓ cup rice malt/brown rice syrup or real maple syrup (maple syrup is sweeter so begin with less)
- ⅓ cup apple cider vinegar (SS) (AA)
- 2 tablespoons flaxseed oil (S) (A)
- handful of chopped chives (optional)

Place the ingredients into a sealable jar and shake well to combine. Shake well before serving. Store the leftovers in the refrigerator. Will last for weeks.

Variation: Maple Dressing (low salicylate, low amine)

Using a blender, mix ⅓ cup of water, ¼ cup of maple syrup, 1 tablespoon of roasted carob powder, 1 tablespoon of sunflower oil or rice bran oil, ¼ teaspoon of quality sea salt and ¼ teaspoon of garlic powder. Place in a sealable jar and store in the refrigerator.

Beetroot Cashew Butter

Makes ½ cup, preparation time 15 minutes

- ½ cup Cashew Butter (H; p. 141)
- 1 medium beetroot, peeled and juiced (you'll need about 5 teaspoons of juice) (S)
- 1 tablespoon real maple syrup
- 2 tablespoons filtered or spring water

Make the Cashew Butter, then place it in a food processor with all the other ingredients and process until combined. You want it to be thick and soft enough for piping onto the popsicles, but not too soft or runny. If needed, thin the mixture by adding an extra teaspoon of maple syrup or water.

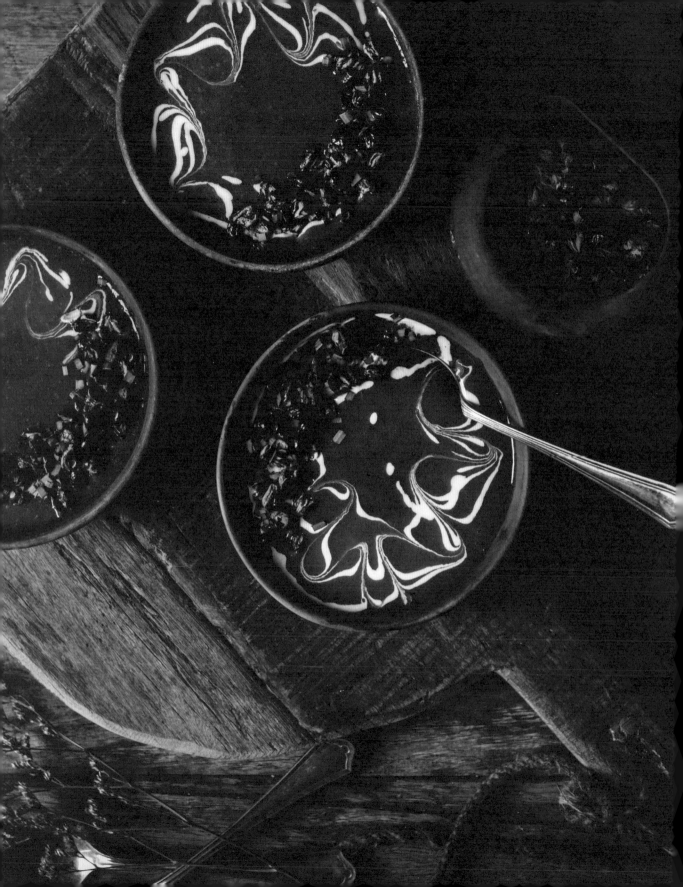

Chapter 13
Lunch and dinner

Beet Detox Soup

Makes 4 bowls, preparation time 15 minutes, cooking time 20 minutes

This liver-loving soup is rich in beta-carotene and betanin, which binds to toxins to allow their safe removal from the body. Top with a splash of Cashew Cream (p. 142) and Roasted Black Beans (p. 131) to make this recipe extra special and totally delicious. To make this recipe paleo, omit the black beans and white potato and use 2 extra cups of diced sweet potato.

- 6 cups filtered or spring water (plus extra)
- 3 large white potatoes (about 2 cups when diced)
- 2 medium sweet potatoes (about 3 cups when diced) (S)
- ½ leek
- ¼–½ teaspoon quality sea salt (begin with ¼ teaspoon)
- 1 teaspoon garlic powder
- 1 medium beetroot, peeled (about ⅔ cup when grated) (S)
- Cashew Cream (p. 142) (H) or White Bean Sauce (p. 146)
- ½ serve Roasted Black Beans (p. 131)
- handful of finely chopped fresh chives to garnish

Place the water in a large pot and bring to the boil. Meanwhile wash, peel and chop the potatoes, sweet potatoes and leek, ensuring you thoroughly wash the leek layers to remove any dirt, and place them into the pot along with the salt and garlic powder. Bring to the boil, cover with a lid and simmer for 20 minutes.

Meanwhile, grate the beetroot and prepare the Cashew Cream if you haven't already made it. To retain the vibrant beet colour do not cook the beets.

Remove the soup from the heat and transfer it to a large mixing bowl, then add 1½ cups of cold filtered or spring water and allow it to cool for 5 minutes, before adding the grated beetroot. Then blend using a stick blender on high (or transfer in batches to a high-speed blender) to make it smooth and creamy.

Serve the soup topped with a drizzle of Cashew Cream, the Roasted Black Beans and fresh chives. I used a squeezie sauce bottle to make a circular pattern with the Cashew Cream and then a toothpick to zigzag across the swirls to create a pattern.

Sweet Potato Flatbread

Makes 12 small flatbreads, preparation and cooking time 1 hour

I am obsessed with this oil-free flatbread recipe — serve them alongside San Choy Bau (p. 159), Lamb Skewers (p. 164) or Cashew Caesar Salad (p. 170), or use them as the base for Asparagus and Black Bean Soft Tacos (p. 155). You can use gluten-free plain/all-purpose flour if you can't eat oat flour (this recipe was tested with oat flour and Bob Mills Gluten-free Baking Flour). You will need a non-stick wok or large non-stick frying pan, rubber spatula, baking (parchment) paper and a rolling pin or long cylinder. You can use any type of cooked sweet potato including roasted, steamed or boiled. These flatbreads can also be used as roti or soft tacos.

- ½ medium sweet potato (about 1 cup of cubed sweet potato) (S)
- 1 cup sweet potato water (reserved from boiling the sweet potato) or filtered or spring water
- 1¼ cups oat flour (or gluten-free plain/all-purpose flour), plus extra for kneading
- ¼ teaspoon quality sea salt

Peel the sweet potato and cut into small cubes. Bring a saucepan of water to the boil and add the sweet potato, then simmer with the lid on for 10 minutes or until soft.

Remove from the heat, strain the liquid into a bowl and reserve 1 cup of the cooking water. Place the sweet potato back into the pot and mash well using a potato masher or a fork. Then mix the mash into the 1 cup of reserved cooking water (you could also use a food processor or high-powered blender for this, but allow the water to cool before using this method).

Meanwhile, heat a non-stick wok or a large frying pan or skillet on medium heat. Before adding the sweet potato mix, place the measured flour and salt nearby, and a rubber/silicon spatula or wooden spoon (don't use metal as it will scratch the pan). Pour the sweet potato mix into the pan, then immediately add the flour and salt and carefully mix using the spatula. Keep scraping the sides and stirring — you want it to form a dough ball. Keep flattening and flipping over the ball until it thickens. Once it becomes a dough ball that is only slightly sticky, remove it from the heat and place it onto a floured chopping board/pastry mat/clean bench. Allow it to cool or wear food prep gloves to knead the dough while warm. While kneading, add about ¼ cup of flour to reduce the stickiness of the ball. Roll into a log and cut it into 8 equal portions. then form each portion into a ball.

Using two large sheets of baking (parchment) paper, place one sheet on the bench and dust with a little flour then flatten one ball in the centre of the paper. Dust with flour then place the other sheet of paper on top (this will allow you to use much less flour when rolling). Roll the first ball into a roundish flatbread, as thin as possible without it splitting (about as thick as a coin). Place a small round bowl or lid (about 12–14 cm/4½–5½ in in diameter) onto the lightly floured dough and cut around it using a knife, to make a round flatbread.

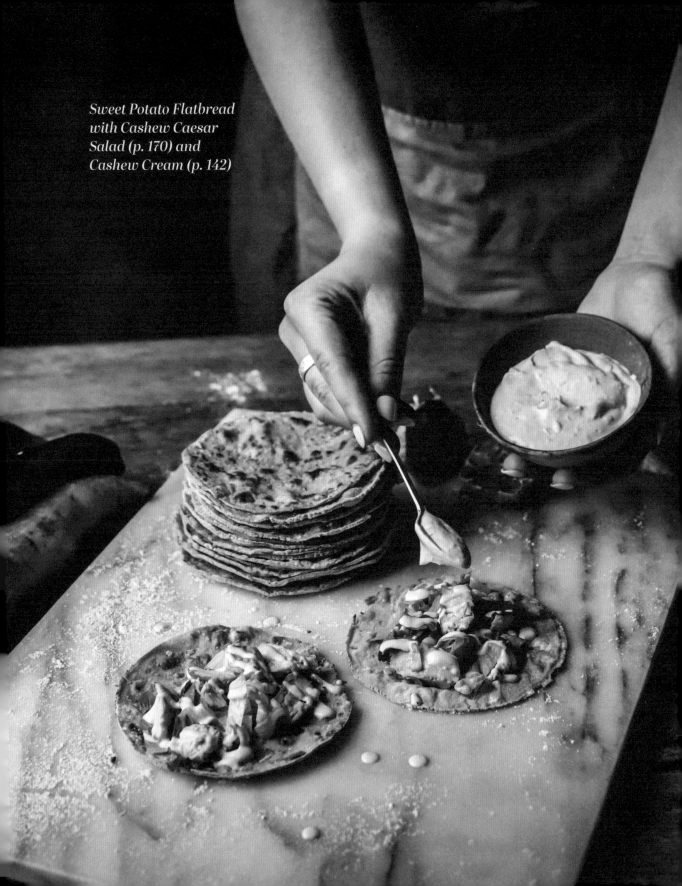

Sweet Potato Flatbread
with Cashew Caesar
Salad (p. 170) and
Cashew Cream (p. 142)

In order to save time, cook the flatbreads as you go (but only cook the ones you want to eat right now). Preheat a medium-sized, non-stick frying pan over moderate–high heat and cook the first flatbread on each side for 2 minutes or until brown spots appear underneath (use a timer). As it's cooking, continue with rolling the next flatbread. When finished, serve with your filling of choice.

Tip: to avoid them going stale, only cook what you need and store the uncooked round flatbreads, separated with baking paper (use the paper you used for rolling) in a sealed container in the refrigerator, and cook them when needed.

Variation: Sweet Potato Chips

Preheat the oven to 180°C (350°F) then make the dough as above. After rolling a large sheet of the dough flat, lift it up via the baking paper and transfer to a large baking tray, then cut it into a grid or triangles and place the tray into the oven. Bake until the chips harden, turning them over after 10 minutes. Ensure they do not burn and remove them individually as they brown to avoid any burning.

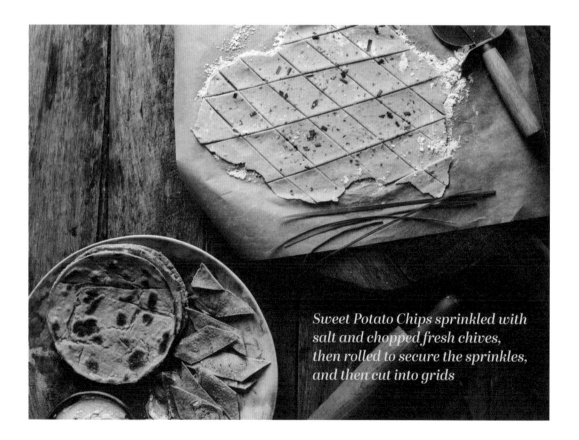

Sweet Potato Chips sprinkled with salt and chopped fresh chives, then rolled to secure the sprinkles, and then cut into grids

Soft Tacos

Makes 8–9 tacos, preparation time 5 minutes, cooking time 10 minutes

Want to make tacos quickly? This simple pancake-like version of soft tacos is a fast and fabulous flatbread alternative to house any type of taco filling. If you have more time to pre-make your tacos, you could make Oat and Leek Flatbread (p. 156) which has a more traditional taco texture — it's just more labour-intensive. You will need a good non-stick frying pan that is not damaged. If you want gluten-free tacos, use chickpea (besan, gram) flour instead of oat flour. Serving suggestions include Asparagus and Black Bean Soft Tacos (p. 155), San Choy Bau (p. 159) and Healthy Fish Tacos (p. 187).

- ¼ cup tapioca starch/flour or arrowroot starch
- 1¼ cups oat flour (G) or chickpea (besan, gram) flour (GF)
- ¼ teaspoon quality sea salt
- 1½ cups filtered or spring water, plus extra
- handful of finely chopped fresh chives (optional)

Combine the two flours and salt in a mixing bowl. Add the water, ½ cup at a time (keep the mixture thick at first to easily mix out the lumps) and mix until smooth, adding extra water if needed for a thin batter. Mix in the chopped chives, if using.

If you use a good non-stick frying pan or skillet you do not need to oil the pan; just ensure the pan is very hot before beginning. When hot, use a ¼ cup to measure the batter and pour it into the middle of the pan, then tilt the pan to spread the batter to make a thin round taco. When the sides of the taco begin to lift off the pan, it is ready to flip over and cook on the other side. If it sticks, your pan is either not hot enough or the taco is undercooked, or the pan is scratched — if this occurs you may need to add a tiny amount of oil to the pan or heat it longer. The batter will thicken in the bowl, making it hard to spread in the pan, so once or twice you may need to add a splash of water into the bowl and mix. Repeat the cooking process and serve the tacos warm.

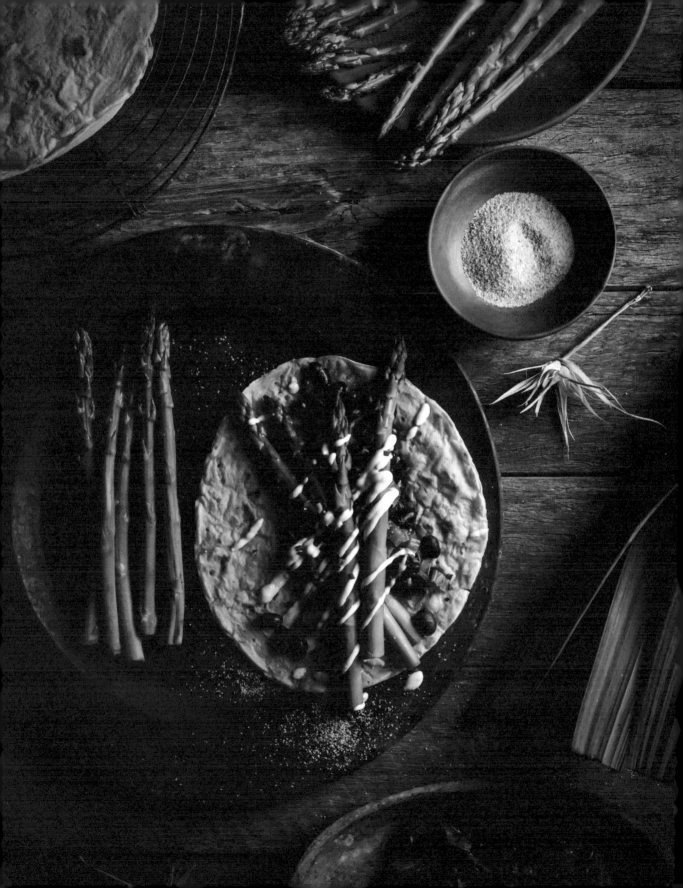

gf   s   veg

Variation: Asparagus and Black Bean Soft Tacos

Makes 6 taco fillings, preparation time 10 minutes, cooking time 10 minutes

Filled with healthy ingredients, your skin and gut will love this nutritious combination of ingredients. Asparagus is an excellent source of quercetin, which is a natural antihistamine. For a quicker meal, choose the Soft Taco recipe (p. 153) or if you have time to roll dough, make the Oat and Leek Flatbread (p. 156) or Sweet Potato Flatbread (p. 150). They are all so good. The gluten-free options are Soft Tacos made with chickpea (besan, gram) flour or either of the flatbread recipes made with gluten-free plain/all-purpose flour.

- 1 bunch fresh asparagus, washed (S)
- 1 x 400 g (14 oz) can organic black beans
- sprinkle of garlic powder (or use 1 small clove garlic)
- 1 serving Caramelized Leek Sauce (p. 142)
- 1 serving flatbread of choice (see above)
- 1 serving Cashew Cream (H) (p. 142) or White Bean Sauce (p. 146)

Cut and discard an inch or more of the stalk end of the asparagus (these are tough to eat), and cut the asparagus in half lengthways so the spears are thin and cook easily. Set aside.

Drain and rinse the black beans and lightly cook them in a non-stick frying pan or skillet on medium heat, along with a sprinkle of the garlic powder. Remove from heat and place them in a covered bowl to keep them warm.

Add 1 tablespoon of filtered or spring water to the pan and place over high heat. Add the asparagus and cook until just soft but still vibrant and green (do not overcook).

Place the leek sauce and beans onto the open tacos, then top with asparagus and drizzle with Cashew Cream.

Oat and Leek Flatbread

Makes 9 flatbreads, preparation and cooking time total 40 minutes

This divine, healing flatbread was my saviour when I had severe food intolerances — it made meals delicious and a little fancy. You can't taste the leeks so it's a great way to get fussy family members enjoying this potent anti-inflammatory vegetable. They can also be used as soft tacos or roti. If you don't have a rolling pin, use any cylinder in your kitchen such as a jar, water bottle or other container.

- ½ cup finely chopped leek (whitest part)
- 1 cup filtered or spring water
- 1¼ cups oat flour (plus about ½ cup for flouring the board) (G)
- ¼ teaspoon quality sea salt

Place the leek into a high-speed blender along with the water. Blend until smooth.

Put the flour and salt in a medium-sized bowl and place the bowl (and a rubber spatula) beside your cooktop for easy reach.

Place the leek mixture into a non-stick wok or a large non-stick frying pan or skillet on high heat, then add the flour and mix well. Continue to mix and scrape down the sides as the dough forms and thickens. The mixture is ready when it resembles a dough ball.

Flour a chopping board, pastry mat or clean benchtop with about ¼ cup of oat flour and place the dough on it to slightly cool, or wear food prep gloves to knead the dough while warm. While kneading, add extra flour (if needed) to reduce the stickiness of the ball. Roll into a log and cut it into 8 equal portions, then form each portion into a ball.

Using two large sheets of baking (parchment) paper, place one sheet on the bench and dust with a little flour then flatten one ball in the centre of the paper. Dust with flour then place the other sheet of paper on top (this will allow you to use much less flour when rolling). Roll the first ball into a roundish flatbread, as thin as possible without it splitting (about as thick as a coin). Place a small round bowl or lid (about 12–14 cm/4½–5½ in in diameter) onto the lightly floured dough and cut around it using a knife, to make a round flatbread.

In order to save time, cook each flatbread as you go (but only cook the ones you want to eat right now). Preheat a medium-sized, non-stick frying pan on moderate–high heat and cook the flatbread on each side for 2 minutes or until brown spots appear underneath (use a timer). As it's cooking, continue with rolling the next flatbread. If there is leftover dough, make a smaller flatbread — you'll be thankful for the extra one as they taste so good. When finished, serve with your filling of choice.

Tip: to avoid them going stale, only cook what you need and store the uncooked round flatbreads, separated with baking paper (use the paper you used for rolling) in a sealed container in the refrigerator, and cook them when needed.

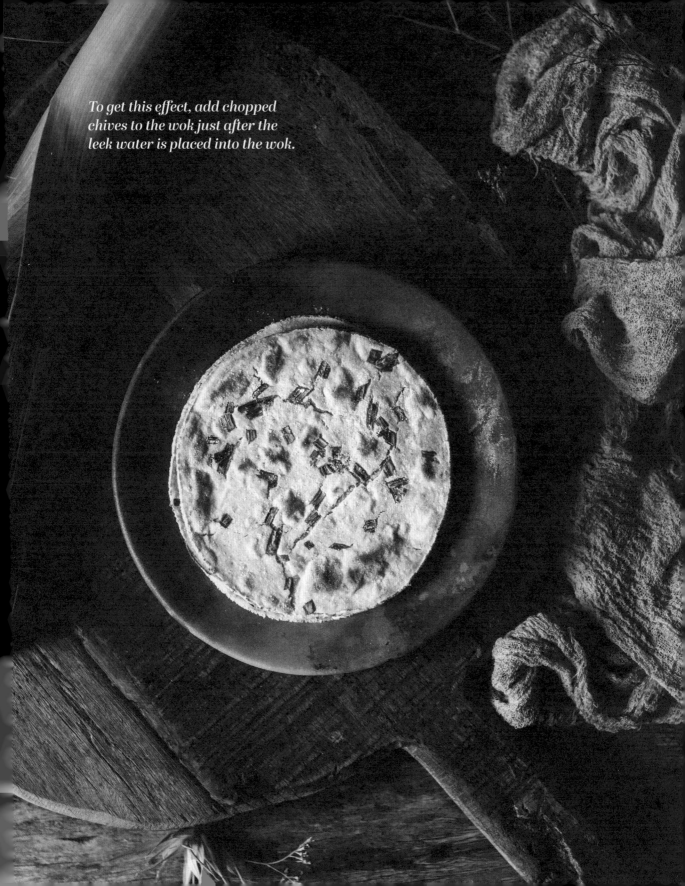

To get this effect, add chopped chives to the wok just after the leek water is placed into the wok.

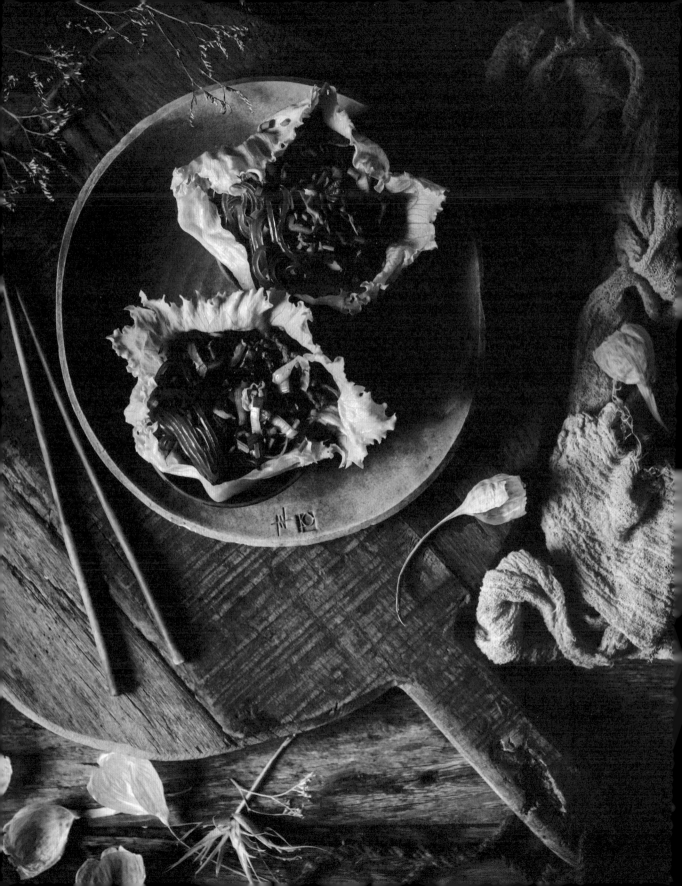

San Choy Bau

Preparation time 10 minutes, cooking time 10 minutes

Lettuce cups are fast food containers for healthy people. This simplified version of San Choy Bau is easy to make, but sometimes your iceberg leaves will separate into absolutely perfect cups and sometimes they will split. That's life. If that happens, make mini/half cups as they work just as well and are even easier to munch into.

If you are following Menu 4 avoid using sweet potato vermicelli for the first three weeks as sweet potato contains salicylates. Vermicelli may not contain salicylates so you can test it on week 4 (it's available from Asian grocers and should only contain sweet potato starch and water so check the ingredients).

- 1 iceberg lettuce (3–4 leaves per person)

The following ingredients are for one person — multiply by the number of people you are cooking for:

- 70 g (2½ oz) sweet potato vermicelli or purple sweet potato vermicelli (available from Asian grocers)
- ¼ leek
- 150 g (5 oz) organic lean beef or lamb mince
- ¼ teaspoon quality sea salt
- 2 spring onions/shallots/scallions (straight stems with no bulb, white and green parts)
- 1 cup finely sliced red cabbage
- handful of mung bean sprouts or pea shoots/sprouts (see p. 33–4)

Wash the iceberg lettuce, trim the stalk and very carefully take apart the leaves. Choose the best leaves for serving and place them onto serving bowls (I use mini dip dishes to hold them upright).

If using vermicelli: bring a saucepan of water to the boil, add the vermicelli and simmer the vermicelli until very soft (about 8 minutes, refer to the packet instructions). Strain in a strainer/colander, rinse with cold water and set aside. Boil some water in a kettle as you will rinse the vermicelli again just before serving.

Next, wash the leek layers to remove any dirt and finely slice. Place a medium-sized non-stick frying pan or skillet on medium heat, add the mince and leek and cook until the meat has completely browned. Sprinkle on the salt, mix then transfer to a bowl.

Rinse the spring onions in water, then thinly slice and set aside. Now rinse the cabbage in water and, using the same pan, lightly sauté the cabbage for 2 minutes (some water should be present to help the sautéing process). Turn off the heat then mix in the spring onions and the cooked mince and stir. Take off the heat and allow it to cool down for a minute, while you rinse the vermicelli in hot water.

Place the mince, vegetables and vermicelli into the lettuce leaf cups, top with sprouts and serve warm.

Vegan Mozzarella

Makes 2 large balls, preparation time 10 minutes, 30 minutes soaking, cooking time 10 minutes

You must try this vegan mozzarella — it's delicious and so easy to make. Cashews are a healthy alternative to cheese and they create a similar texture to dairy mozzarella. Serve it with Quinoa Nourish Bowl (p. 166) or salads such as Cashew Caesar Salad (p. 170).

- 1 cup raw cashews (not roasted or salted) (H)
- 4 teaspoons tapioca starch/flour
- 1 small clove garlic, peeled and crushed (or 1 teaspoon garlic powder)
- ¾ teaspoon quality sea salt
- ½ teaspoon citric acid or ascorbic acid
- ½ cup filtered or spring water

Soak the cashews in boiling hot water for 20–30 minutes (or if you have time, place them in a bowl of water in the refrigerator overnight). Drain the cashews and rinse well, then add them to a high-speed blender with the other ingredients and blend until smooth.

Place a good quality non-stick frying pan or skillet on medium heat and scoop half of the mixture into the pan. Using a rubber spatula (as metal will damage your pan), stir the mixture continuously, scraping down the sides to ensure the mixture does not overly stick to the pan. After about a minute, the mixture will start to thicken. Continue to quickly stir and fold the mozzarella, working it into a ball. This whole process will take about 5 minutes, so after the ball has formed, scrape down the sides, roll the mozzarella into a solid ball then place it onto a plate to cool down.

Rinse and dry the pan, then place it back onto the heat to cook the next mozzarella ball. Repeat the process. Once cooled, the balls can be put into a container with the lid on and placed in the refrigerator for at least an hour. We used plastic wrap to mould the mozzarella into a traditional mozzarella shape, by twisting the top tightly (see image).

Once they are cold and firm, the balls can be sliced (or pulled apart) and added to pizzas, pasta, toast, salads or snack on it with carrot and celery sticks.

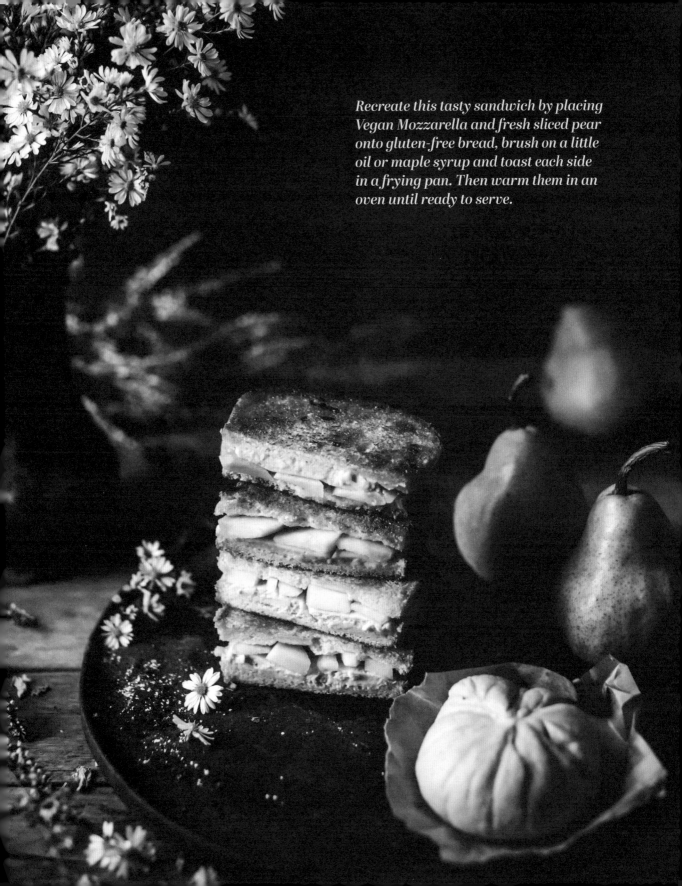

Recreate this tasty sandwich by placing
Vegan Mozzarella and fresh sliced pear
onto gluten-free bread, brush on a little
oil or maple syrup and toast each side
in a frying pan. Then warm them in an
oven until ready to serve.

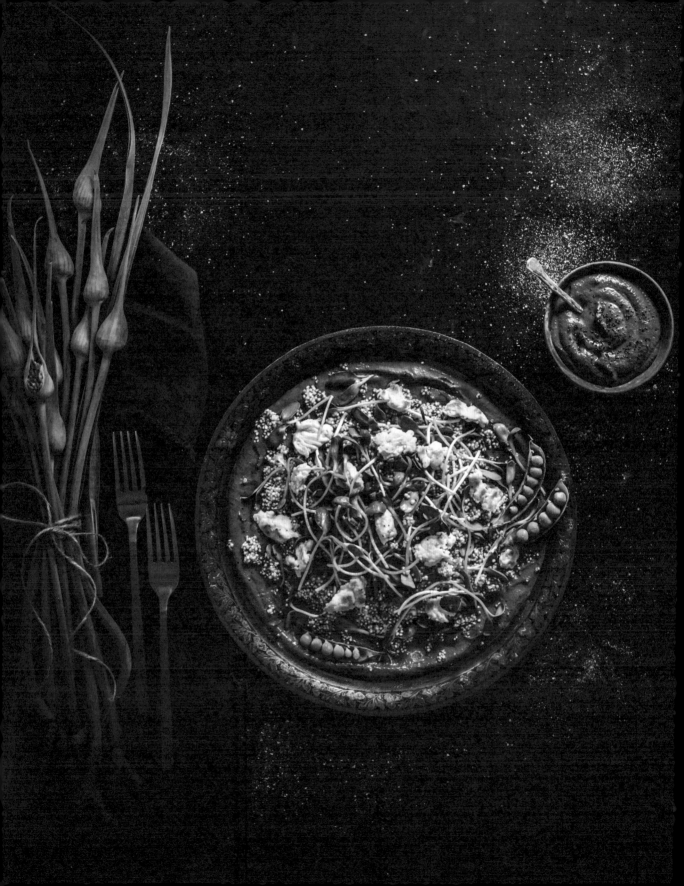

Quinoa and Chicken Salad with Beet Cream

Makes 2 servings, preparation time 20 minutes, cooking time 20 minutes

This tasty dish is rich in skin-firming protein, gut-loving fibre and alkalizing sprouts and beetroot, which help to improve blood flow to your skin.

- 1 cup white quinoa
- 2 cups filtered or spring water
- handful of sugar snap peas (S)
- 2 cups sunflower or pea shoots/sprouts (S)
- 350 g (12 oz) chicken mince (preferably organic or free range)
- ¼ teaspoon quality sea salt
- poppy seeds to garnish (optional)

For the Beet Cream:
- ½ cup raw cashews (soaked in hot water for 20 minutes) (H)
- 2½ tablespoons finely grated beetroot (S)
- ¼ teaspoon quality sea salt
- 1 fresh clove garlic, crushed, or 1 teaspoon of garlic powder
- ½ cup filtered or spring water

Rinse the quinoa in water, drain and place it into a medium saucepan with the water (you need 1 part quinoa to 2 parts water). Put on the lid and bring to the boil, then remove the lid and simmer. Check often to ensure the quinoa does not boil dry or burn. Once the water has reduced and the quinoa is nearly cooked (about 10 minutes), turn off the heat, cover with a lid and set aside to continue steaming for another 5 minutes. Do not overcook.

Meanwhile, rinse and halve the sugar snap peas, rinse the sprouts and set aside.

To prepare the Beet Cream, drain the cashews and add the grated beetroot, salt, garlic and water to a high-speed blender and blend until smooth. Set aside.

Cook the mince in a medium-sized non-stick frying pan or skillet on moderate heat, until lightly browned and cooked through (ensure there is no pink). Season with salt and briefly mix.

On two large plates, spread the Beet Cream onto the bottom of the dish, then top with the quinoa, chicken, sprouts and peas. Sprinkle with poppy seeds if using.

Lamb Skewers

Serves 2, preparation time 20 minutes, cooking time 15 minutes

Lamb Skewers are a tasty, protein-rich meal which supplies iron for healthy blood, selenium for liver health and zinc for healthy skin, hair and nails. For a larger main meal, you can serve the skewers with Oat and Leek Flatbread (p. 156) or for an easy paleo option, make the Sweet Potato Boats recipe on p. 180. To make this a low salicylate/amine meal (for Menu 4), omit the cashew cream and zucchini (courgette) and use sautéed leeks instead. If you cannot buy lamb chunks, buy any type of quality lamb or beef steaks and dice it yourself into 2 cm (1 in) pieces — it's easy with a good carving knife. You will need 6 skewers.

- 2 medium zucchinis/courgettes (SS)
- 400 g (14 oz) diced lamb chunks such as lamb steaks, lamb backstrap or topside (preferably grass-fed or organic)
- quality sea salt to taste
- 3 cups finely sliced iceberg lettuce
- 1 cup shredded red cabbage
- ¼ cup fresh chives, finely sliced
- 1 serving White Bean Sauce (p. 146) or Cashew Cream (p. 142), premade (H)

If you are using wooden skewers for the lamb, soak them in water for a few minutes as this will prevent the skewers from burning under the grill.

Preheat the grill to 190°C (375°F) or high heat, and cover the base of the grill tray with foil (optional, to catch the fat and reduce cleaning time).

Wash the zucchinis and slice them so each piece is approximately the same size as the lamb chunks (about 2 cm/1 in wide).

Thread the lamb chunks and zucchini onto the skewers, alternating each one (as shown in the photo) and lightly season them with a sprinkle of salt, if desired. Place the skewers under the grill until the meat is lightly brown on each side (check often to avoid burning). Turn approximately every 4 minutes. Once cooked, remove from the grill and place on serving plates.

While the skewers are cooking, mix together the lettuce, red cabbage and chives, and place a pile of the salad onto each serving plate. Remove the lamb skewers from the grill and add them to the plates, then drizzle the Cashew Cream onto the raw vegetables.

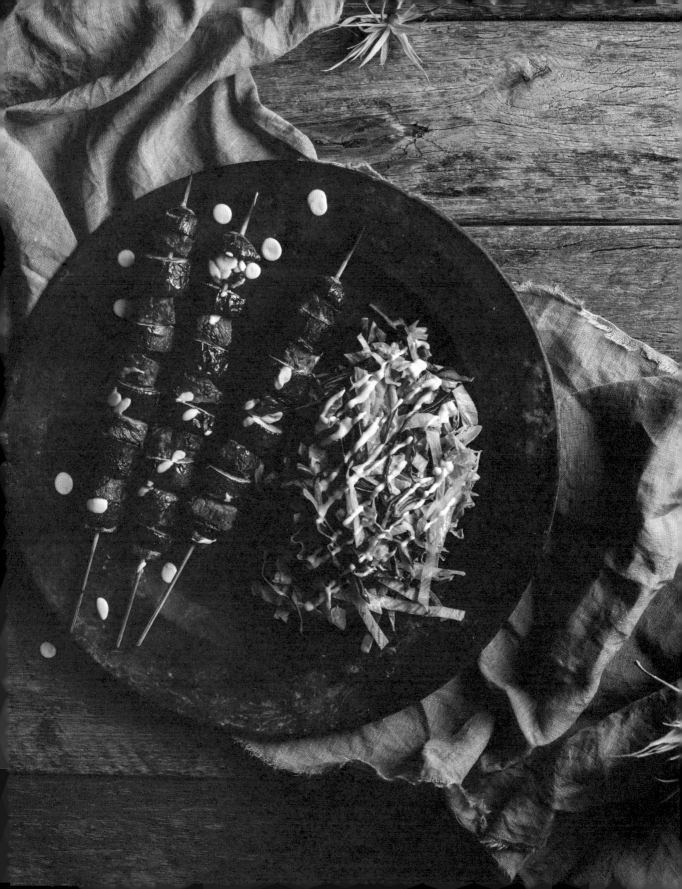

Quinoa Nourish Bowl

Serves 2, preparation time 30 minutes, cooking time 45 minutes

Whether you call it a nourish, poke or buddha bowl, this skin-friendly meal offers a powerhouse of nutrients, fibre and protein, and it tastes great too. Nourish bowls were invented to use up leftovers, so you do not need to use every element in this recipe — use what you have. I love this topped with Cashew Cream or White Bean Sauce, as it makes the zucchini pasta creamy; or try Omega Salad Dressing (p. 147) with chives for a vinaigrette.

- 2–4 baby beets/beetroots, whole (S)
- ½ x 400 g (14 oz) can organic chickpeas (garbanzo beans), drained and rinsed
- oil of choice (refer to 'Cooking oil options for your skin type', p. 92)
- quality sea salt, to taste
- 1 small–medium sweet potato, peeled and sliced into round discs (S)
- ½ cup uncooked red or white quinoa
- 1 cup filtered or spring water
- 1 serving Vegan Mozzarella (p. 160) (H) or 2 chicken thigh fillets, sliced
- 1 medium zucchini/courgette (SS)
- ½ cup finely sliced red cabbage
- fresh chives, finely chopped, or pea shoots/sprouts (p. 33), to garnish
- Cashew Cream (p. 142), White Bean Sauce (p. 146) or Omega Salad Dressing (p. 147)

Preheat the oven to 200°C (400°F) and line a baking tray with a silicon mat or baking (parchment) paper and set aside.

You can boil, steam or roast the baby beets. First, wash and scrub the beets then, if roasting, place the beets onto a tray and cover with a little oil (you will peel the beets after roasting). Cook in the oven for about 45 minutes or until soft.

Place the chickpeas into a pot or container that has a lid, coat with 1 teaspoon of oil (if using), sprinkle on salt, close the lid and shake lightly to evenly coat the chickpeas. Then place the chickpeas and sweet potato onto the same baking tray as the beets — these ingredients will take 30 minutes to cook, so add them to the beet tray 15 minutes after the beets have been placed into the oven.

To cook the quinoa, rinse with water in a fine sieve then place into a pot with the water. Cover with a lid and bring to the boil, then remove the lid and turn to a low heat, which will allow for a light simmer. Once the water has reduced and the quinoa is just cooked turn the heat off, cover with the lid and set aside to continue steaming for another 5 minutes.

Meanwhile, cook the chicken if you are using it instead of mozzarella. If using chicken, salt the chicken and pan fry it on medium–high heat until thoroughly cooked through and nicely browned.

Now prepare the zucchini. Rinse it and cut off each end. The zucchini noodles can be made with a vegetable spiralizer (like we did in the photo) or use a basic vegetable peeler to create a long, flat noodle shape. Remember to check on the vegetables and chickpeas throughout the cooking process to ensure they do not overcook.

Remove the mozzarella from the refrigerator and slice it into 1 cm (⅓ in) thick slices. You can briefly fry the slices in a pan on low heat to make it look like haloumi. Remove the vegetables from the oven and peel the beets. Assemble all the ingredients into two large, wide bowls, top with chives or pea shoots and serve alongside your dressing of choice.

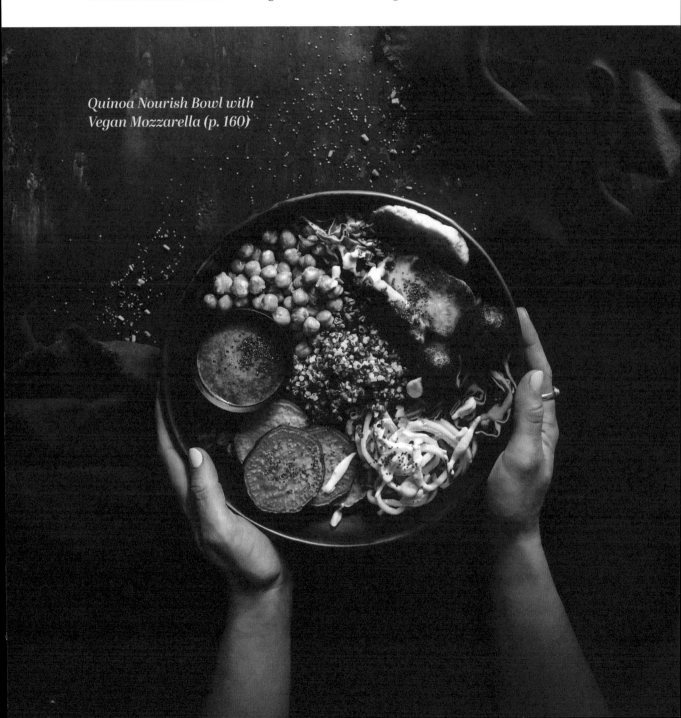

Quinoa Nourish Bowl with Vegan Mozzarella (p. 160)

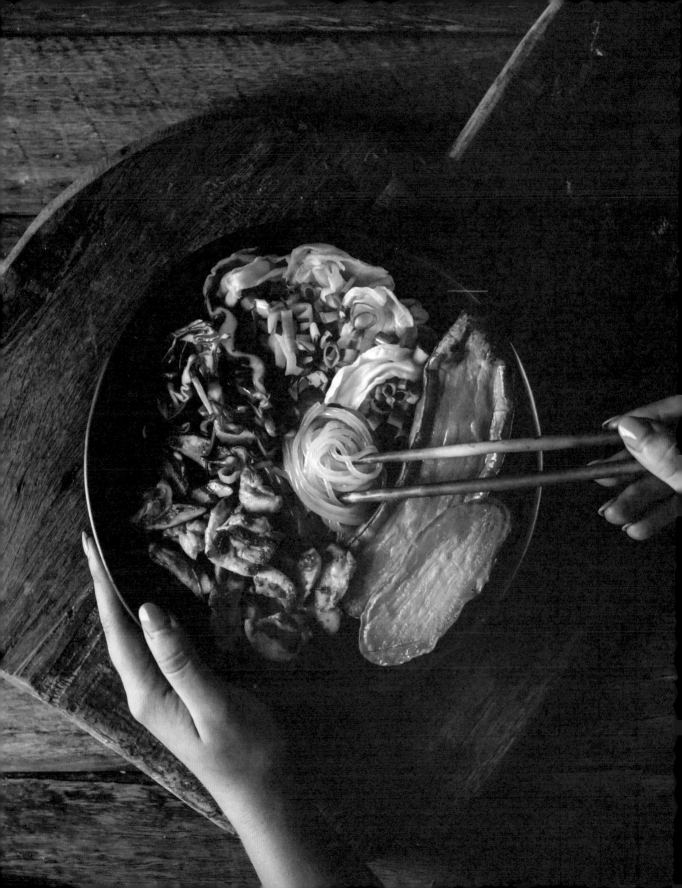

Sweet Potato Nourish Bowl

Serves 2, preparation time 15 minutes, cooking time 45 minutes

I think nourish bowls were invented to give leftovers a delicious name. In this dish, I used leftover caramelized leeks and Sweet Potato Boats, and teamed them with fresh vegetables, chicken and sweet potato vermicelli, which is made from nothing but sweet potato starch and water (from Asian grocers; check ingredients before purchase as some contain wheat). If you are vegan, sub the chicken for Roasted Chickpeas (p. 131). If you want a creamy dressing, Cashew Cream (p. 142) or White Bean Sauce (p. 146) go brilliantly and can be prepared while the sweet potato roasts in the oven.

- 1 medium sweet potato, scrubbed and halved lengthways (S)
- oil (refer to 'Cooking oil options for your skin type', p. 92)
- 1 handful sweet potato vermicelli (S)
- 2 skinless chicken thigh fillets (preferably organic or free range)
- fresh chives, washed and finely sliced (optional)
- 1 cup finely sliced red cabbage, washed
- ½ cup finely sliced leeks, layers washed thoroughly
- fresh spring onions (scallions, shallots), washed and finely sliced (optional)

Preheat the oven to 200°C (400°F) and line a baking tray with a silicon mat or baking (parchment) paper. Place the sweet potato halves onto the mat. Place a teaspoon of oil onto the palm of your hand, then massage the oil into the sweet potato on all sides. Roast the sweet potato for 45–60 minutes or until very soft.

Meanwhile, make your sauce of choice.

Next, cook the vermicelli. Bring a large pot of water to the boil then place the vermicelli into the pot, and stir occasionally, simmering for at least 8 minutes (refer to packet instructions).

Slice the chicken into strips. Heat a large non-stick frying pan or skillet on medium–high heat. You do not need oil, as the chicken has enough fat to self-oil the pan. Cook the chicken until golden and cooked through, adding fresh chopped chives if desired. Remove from the pan, then lightly fry the red cabbage, leek and spring onions (if using) in the chicken juices (the water from the washed vegetables should make a sauce when stirred).

Place the sweet potato, vermicelli and chicken into serving bowls. Then add the red cabbage, leeks and spring onions and drizzle on your sauce of choice.

Cashew Caesar Salad

Serves 2, preparation time 30 minutes (including soaking time), cooking time 15 minutes

I love this simple recipe, which is a (much) healthier version of the Caesar salads you'll find in your average restaurant or café. It's delicious too. If you are vegan or vegetarian you can substitute the chicken with Roasted Chickpeas (p. 131) or Vegan Mozzarella (p. 160). If you are following Menu 4, use iceberg lettuce instead of cos (romaine) and make White Bean Sauce (p. 146) instead of Cashew Cream. Use a squeezie sauce bottle to get a picture-perfect drizzle.

- 2 chicken thighs, preferably organic or free range
- 2 baby cos (romaine) lettuces (or ½ iceberg lettuce if on Menu 4)
- handful of fresh chives, washed
- 2 slices gluten-free bread of choice (omit if on Menu 4; use crushed cashews if paleo)
- garlic powder or 1 clove garlic, finely chopped
- sprinkle of quality sea salt (less than ¼ teaspoon)
- 1 serving Cashew Cream (H), p. 142 (or White Bean Sauce, p. 146)

Chop the chicken into thin strips, wash the individual lettuce leaves, and finely chop the chives, and set aside.

Toast the bread and slice into croutons, or you can lightly pulse in a high-speed blender to create course breadcrumbs (like we did for the photo). Set aside.

Season the chicken with garlic and salt. Place a medium-sized non-stick frying pan or skillet on moderate heat and cook the chicken on all sides until lightly browned and cooked through then set aside.

Meanwhile, chop the lettuce into strips and place it into bowls. Arrange the chicken on top of the lettuce, top it with your homemade croutons/breadcrumbs and chives and drizzle with Cashew Cream or White Bean Sauce.

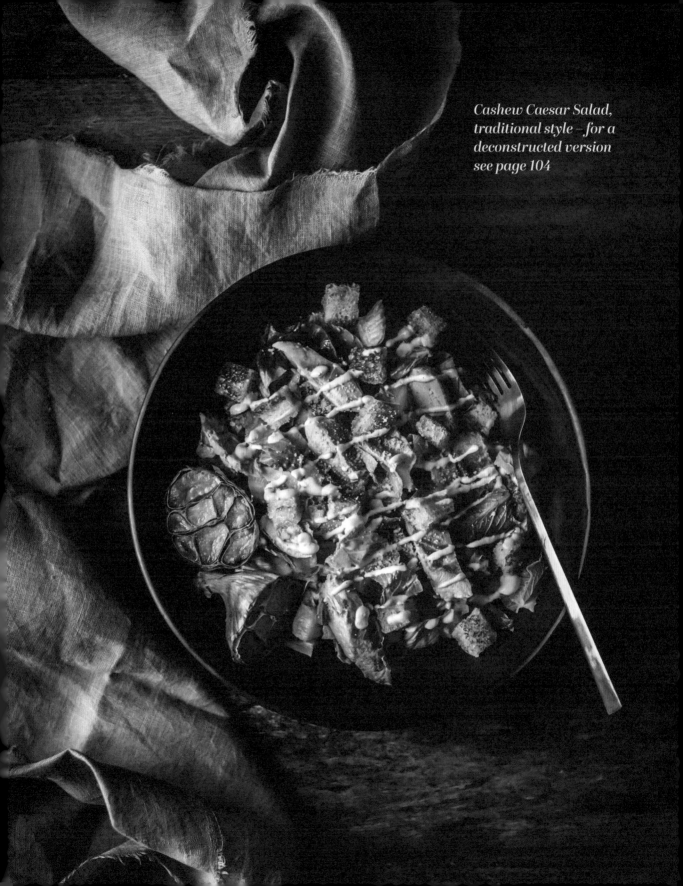

Cashew Caesar Salad,
traditional style – for a
deconstructed version
see page 104

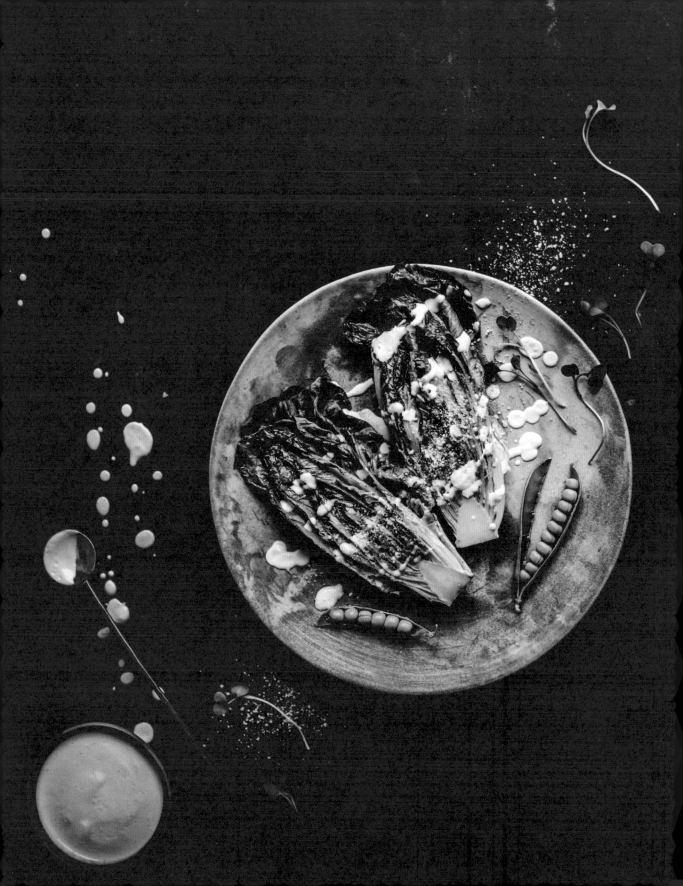

Charred Cos Lettuce

Serves 2 as a side salad, preparation time 5 minutes, cooking time 5 minutes

Who knew charred lettuce was a thing ... it tastes so good. Serve this in your Nourish Bowl (pp. 166-9) or with chicken, fish or lamb (anything, really). This lettuce is delicious on its own — thanks to the maple syrup — but you can omit the maple syrup and drizzle it with Cashew Cream (p. 142) for a sugar-free wow factor.

- 2 whole baby cos (romaine) lettuces (S), washed and halved lengthwise
- 1 teaspoon real maple syrup (or oil of choice if not using maple syrup: refer to 'Cooking oil options for your skin type', p. 92)

Heat a large non-stick frying pan or skillet on medium heat, add a teaspoon of maple syrup or your oil of choice and add the lettuce, flat side down, to brown on the side that has been cut. Serve warm.

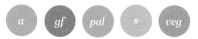

Crispy Sweet Potato Gnocchi

Serves 2, preparation time 60 minutes, cooking time 30 minutes

Thank me later. Golden and crispy on the outside, and warm and gooey on the inside, just how a good — no, great — gnocchi should be.

- 1 cup raw cashews (H)
- 2 medium sweet potatoes (S), scrubbed (about 1½ cups when mashed)
- ½ cup tapioca starch or arrowroot starch
- 1 teaspoon garlic powder
- ¾–1 teaspoon quality sea salt
- oil of choice (refer to 'Cooking oil options for your skin type', p. 92)
- ½–1 serving Cashew Cream (p. 142)

Serving suggestion:
- ½ cup red cabbage, washed and finely sliced
- 4 large zucchinis/courgettes, spiralized or sliced into thin noodles (SS)
- fresh chives, washed and finely sliced

If you have not already made the Cashew Cream, soak 1 cup of cashews in hot water and set aside. Line 2 large baking trays with baking (parchment) paper and set aside.

Bring a medium pot of water to the boil. Peel and cube the sweet potato, then add to the pot and boil until soft (about 15 minutes). Drain, then remove excess water with paper towels or a clean tea towel. Set aside to cool.

Next, place the cup of raw cashews into a high-speed blender and pulse until the mixture resembles breadcrumbs or flour (do not excessively blend as it will turn into nut butter), then add the tapioca starch, garlic powder and salt, and briefly blend. Set aside.

Place the sweet potato in a large flat-based bowl and mash, then stir ¼ cup of the cashew flour mix into the mash. Add another ¼ cup of flour and kneed together until the flour is well mixed in. Add the remaining flour as needed. The dough may be slightly sticky. Wrap the dough in some plastic wrap and place in the refrigerator to firm for about 10 minutes.

While the dough is firming make the Cashew Cream if you haven't already, and set aside in the refrigerator. Remove the dough and separate into three balls, and place one onto the lined baking tray. Roll it into a long snake-like piece about 1 cm (⅓ in) wide and then cut into gnocchi-sized pieces, about 1 x 2 cm ⅓ x 1 in). Press individual pieces down lightly with a fork to make a pattern on the top. Repeat with the other two balls of dough, then set aside and leave to firm (about 10 minutes).

While the gnocchi is firming, make the zucchini noodles with a vegetable spiralizer or peel zucchini strips to create a large, flat noodle shapes. Set aside.

Place a large non-stick pan or skillet on medium heat with a dash of oil and add half of the gnocchi to the pan, cooking until lightly browned (about 1–2 minutes on each side). Remove from the pan and set aside while you cook the rest of the gnocchi.

Once the gnocchi is ready, add the zucchini noodles and cabbage to the frying pan and heat for 1 minute, then place onto a serving dish or into two bowls. Drizzle with Cashew Cream, then place the gnocchi on top and sprinkle with chives.

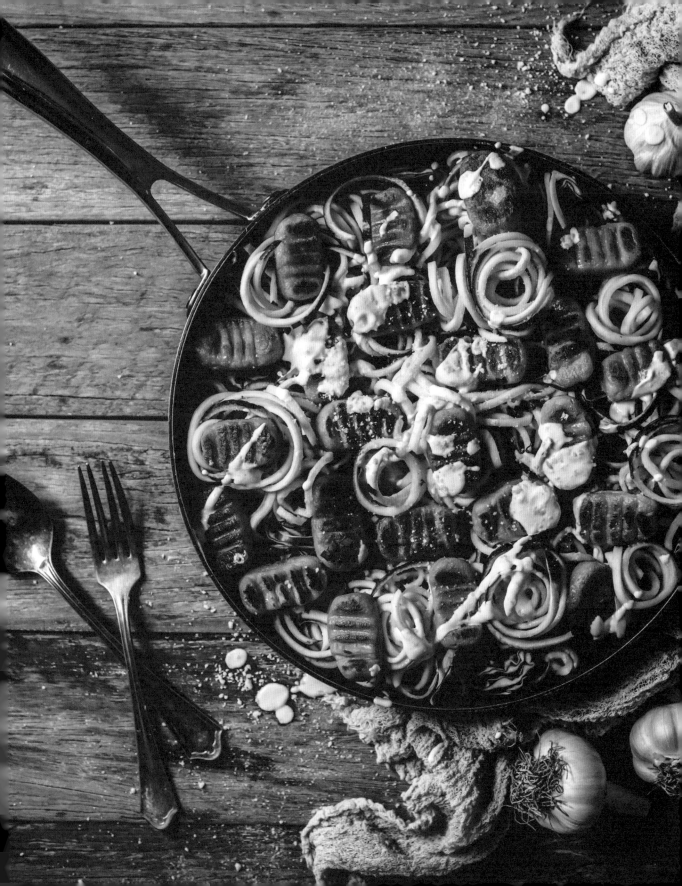

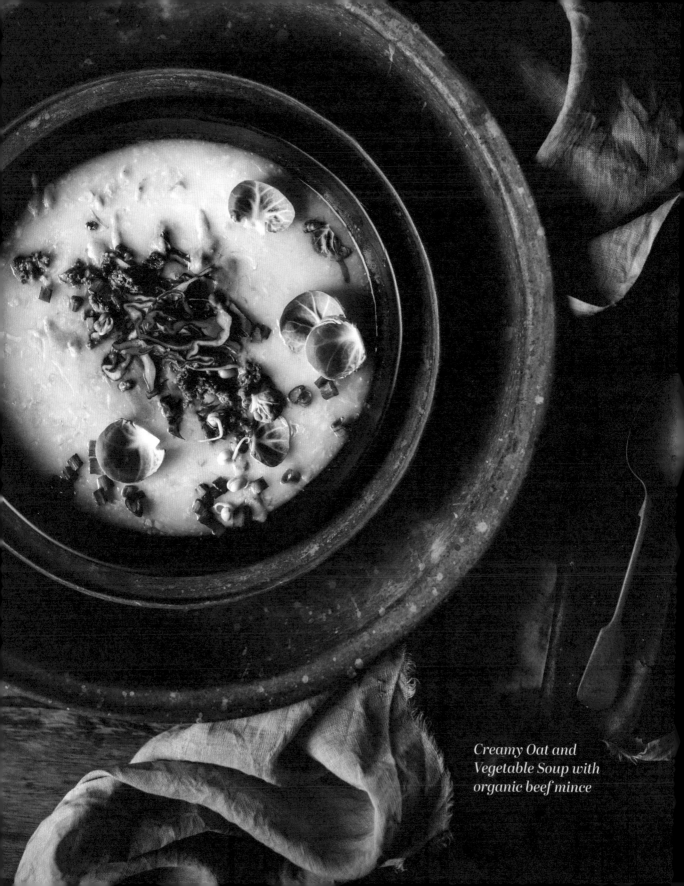

Creamy Oat and Vegetable Soup with organic beef mince

Creamy Oat and Vegetable Soup

Serves 2–3 (or one hungry adult), preparation time 10 minutes, cooking time 15 minutes

Who knew oat soup was a thing?! Oats make a lovely, creamy and thick soup. This is one of my favourite healthy recipes, which I heavily relied on while healing my immune system issues. To save time (and create a creamier soup), you can let the oats and vegetables soak in the water and cook it later, when you get home in the evening. If you are paleo-minded, skip the oats and add extra vegetables. If you have amine/histamine intolerance, add the cooked meat directly to your serving bowl, not the soup pot, so if there are leftovers they are meat-free (cook your meat fresh each day).

- 1 cup rolled oats (or ½ cup if cooking for 1)
- 10 cups filtered or spring water (5 cups if cooking for 1 person)
- ¼ leek
- 4 small Brussels sprouts, stalk end trimmed (use 2 if cooking for one person)
- 2 cups white cabbage, very finely sliced
- ½ cup finely shredded red cabbage
- ¼ teaspoon quality sea salt (or to taste, but don't overdo it!)
- 2 large spring onions (shallots, scallions), finely chopped

Protein choices:
- 200 g (7 oz) organic/free range chicken tenderloins or thigh fillets, thinly chopped, or 180 g (6 oz) organic lean beef or chicken mince (150 g/5 oz if cooking for one person). If you are vegan opt for 1 cup of Roasted Black Beans (p. 131) instead of meat.

Bake the Roasted Black Beans now (if using the vegan option).

Place the oats and the water into a large pot and bring to the boil. You can partially cover the pot with a lid but it will boil over if fully covered.

Meanwhile, prepare the vegetables. Rinse the leek to remove any dirt from the layers, finely chop and add to the soup pot. Remove the outer leaves of the Brussels sprouts, as these look nice on the soup and you can add them for decoration when serving (refer to the image). Finely slice the remaining portion of Brussels sprouts and place into the soup pot. Place the white cabbage in the pot and cook for 10–15 minutes. If you prefer your red cabbage cooked, you can add it to the pot now, for the last few minutes of cooking; otherwise it will be added last.

Meanwhile heat a good non-stick frying pan or skillet on high heat and cook the meat (do not add oil, as the meat will self-oil the pan), sprinkle half the salt onto the meat to season it and cook thoroughly on all sides until browned.

Sprinkle the remaining salt into the soup pot and mix. Turn off the heat and stir in the spring onions. Ladle the soup into large soup bowls and top with meat (or black beans), Brussels sprout leaves and raw red cabbage. If using meat, after removing the meat from the frying pan you can make a gravy with the juices by turning up the heat and adding a ladleful (about ⅓ cup) of soup into the pan, then mix vigorously with a plastic spatula. Top the soup with the gravy, as shown in the image.

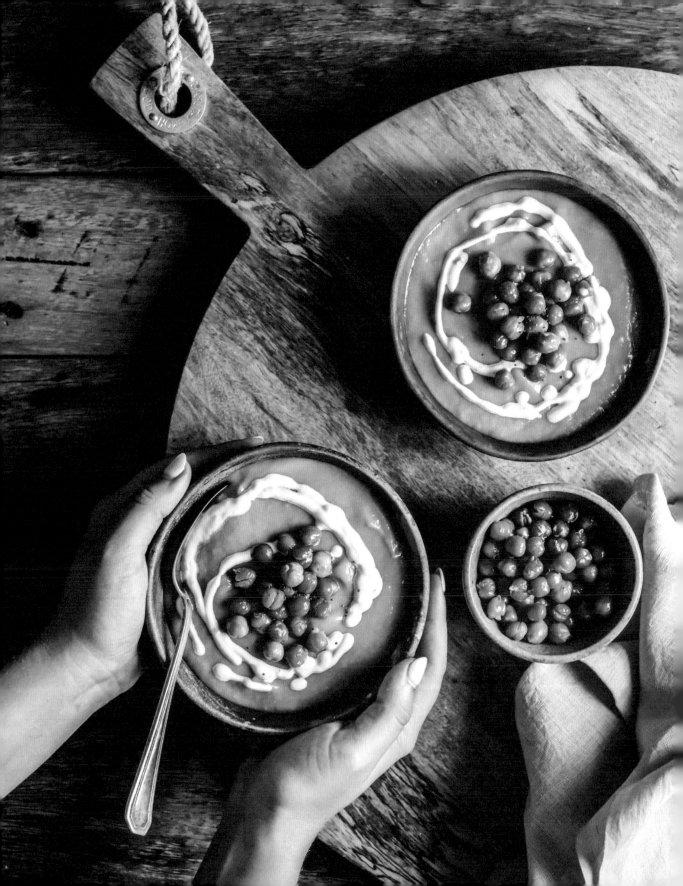

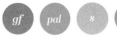

Green Detox Soup

Serves 2, preparation time 15 minutes, cooking time 20 minutes

Brussels sprouts and white potato have fantastic detoxifying abilities thanks to their rich content of glutathione. Brussels sprouts have the added benefit of supplying omega-3 for anti-inflammatory support. Leeks are anti-inflammatory and alkalizing, which can be beneficial for those with skin inflammation. You can decorate this soup with Cashew Cream (p. 142) and Roasted Chickpeas (p. 131) or Roasted Black Beans (p. 131), and you can make it paleo by omitting the potatoes. Make this soup low salicylate and suitable for Menu 4 by omitting the asparagus and replacing it with white cabbage; do not use Cashew Cream, and avoid potato if needed.

- 5–6 cups filtered or spring water
- 1¼ cups white potato, peeled and diced
- 1¼ cups Brussels sprouts, ends trimmed and quartered
- 1 cup asparagus, ends trimmed and roughly chopped (S)
- 1 cup leek, washed and finely diced
- 1 cup diced celery
- 1–3 cloves garlic, crushed or chopped (or 2 teaspoons garlic powder)
- ¼–½ teaspoon quality sea salt
- ½ bunch fresh chives, finely chopped, plus extra to serve
- ½ serving Roasted Chickpeas (p. 131) or Roasted Black Beans (optional, p. 131)
- Cashew Cream (H) (optional, p. 142)

Place the water in a large pot and bring to the boil, then add the potatoes, Brussels sprouts, asparagus, leek, celery, garlic and salt. Cover with a lid, bring back to the boil then reduce to a simmer. Top up with water during the cooking process if needed, and boil for 20 minutes.

Remove from the heat and allow to slightly cool. Then pour the soup into a high-speed blender and add the chives. This can be done in two batches, depending on the size of the blender. Blend until smooth. Taste and add more salt and garlic if desired. Pour into a bowl and decorate, if desired, with Roasted Chickpeas, Cashew Cream and chives.

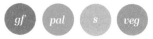

Sweet Potato Boats

Makes 6 boats, preparation time 30 minutes, cooking time 45 minutes

Ahoy, get your sexy sea legs into shape with this super sweet potato recipe. To make the perfect drizzle, use a squeezie sauce bottle and test run on an empty plate until you have perfected your zig zag. Make six and save them for snacks, or prep a meal for two people. Savour them on their own or with a side salad. To make this paleo, omit the beans.

- 3 medium sweet potatoes (choose ones with similar size and shape) (S)
- 1 teaspoon oil of choice (refer to 'Cooking oil options for your skin type', p. 92)
- Cashew Cream (H) (p. 142) or White Bean Sauce (p. 146)
- 1 x 400 g (14 oz) can organic black beans (paleo option: 300 g/10½ oz organic beef/chicken/lamb mince)
- ½ teaspoon garlic powder (optional)
- 2 spring onions (scallions/shallots),washed and finely sliced
- handful of chopped fresh chives or mung bean sprouts (p. 34), to garnish
- quality sea salt to taste (optional)

Preheat the oven to 200°C (400°F) and line a baking tray with a silicon mat or baking (parchment) paper.

Wash and scrub the sweet potatoes, cut them in half lengthways, place them onto the tray and sparingly rub oil onto each one. Bake for 45 minutes or until soft.

If you have not done so already, prepare the Cashew Cream or White Bean Sauce and set aside.

Drain the black beans and rinse in water. Place a medium-sized frying pan or skillet on medium heat, then add the black beans. Sprinkle on the garlic powder (if using) and lightly cook the beans (or meat) for about 4 minutes or until cooked through, gently stirring a few times. Stir in the spring onions, turn off the heat and set aside.

Remove the sweet potatoes from the oven then use a spoon to scoop out the middle of each sweet potato half so it is hollow like a canoe. Save the leftover sweet potato to use in wraps (Oat and Leek Flatbread, p. 156) or salads. Fill the boats with the bean mix, drizzle on the sauce and garnish with chives or sprouts, and a pinch of salt if desired.

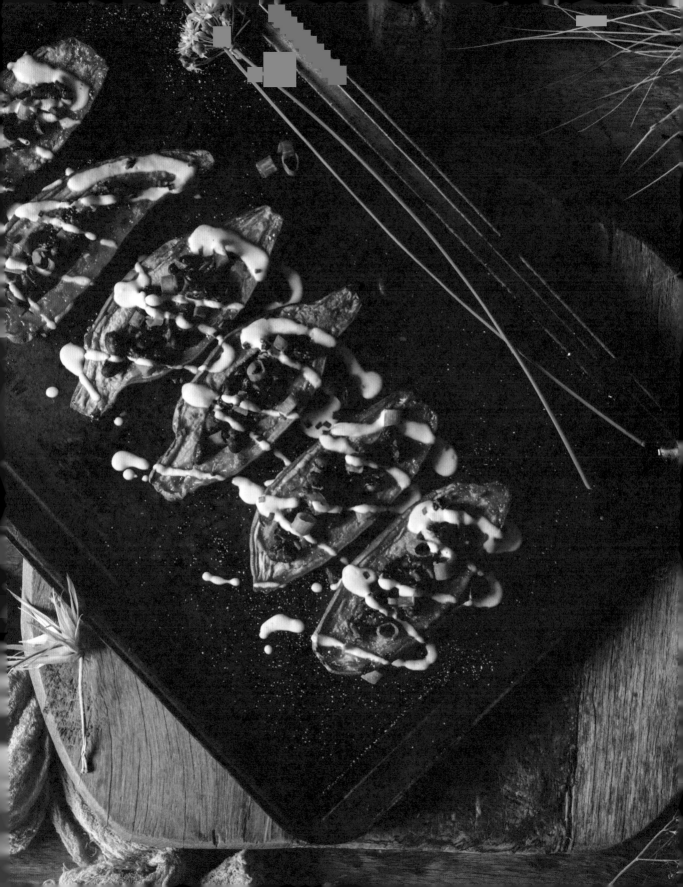

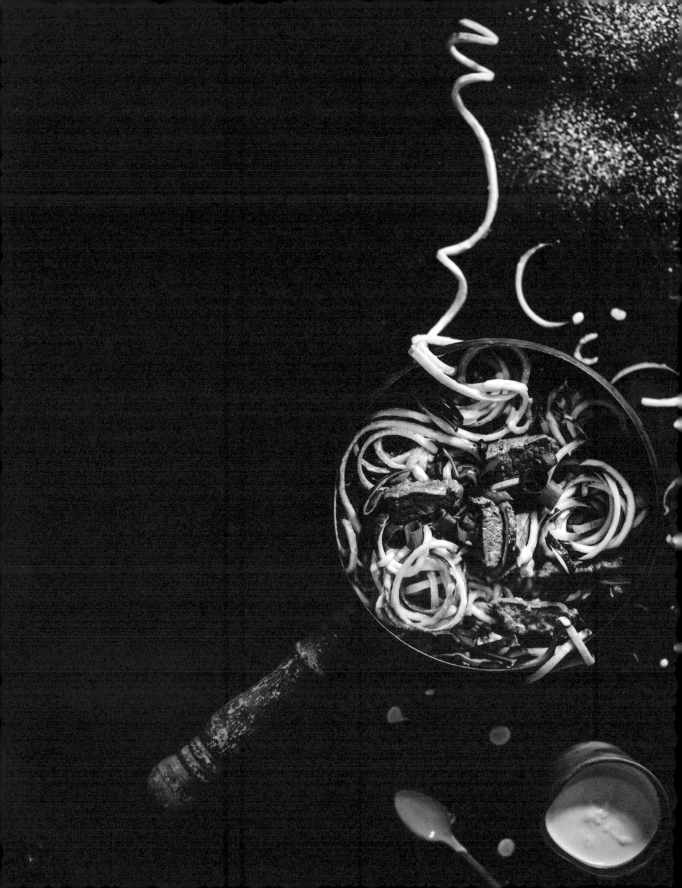

Lamb and Zucchini Pasta

Serves 2, preparation time 20 minutes, cooking time 10 minutes

Say hello to the healthiest pasta in the world — zucchini (courgette) noodles are unprocessed and fresh, and they taste fabulous. You don't even need a spiralizing gadget to make the noodles — simply use a potato peeler and in less than 5 minutes you have homemade pasta that your waistline will looove (flat belly on the way, I promise).

If you can't consume cashews try Vegan Mayo, White Bean Sauce (p. 146) or another condiment from the book: there is a friendly alternative for everything!

- 1 serving of Cashew Cream (H) (this is the paleo option, p. 142) or Vegan Mayo (p. 146)
- ¼ cup red cabbage
- ¼ cup sliced spring onions (shallots, scallions), roots trimmed
- 4 large zucchinis (courgettes), washed (peeled if desired) (SS)
- 300 g (10½ oz) lamb backstrap, beef or lamb strips (preferably organic or grass fed)
- handful of fresh chives, finely chopped
- ½ teaspoon quality sea salt

Make the Cashew Cream or your sauce of choice.

Wash the vegetables and thinly slice the red cabbage and set aside. Trim the ends of the zucchini. To make spaghetti-shaped noodles, use a vegetable spiralizer (like we did for the photograph), or create wide, flat fettuccini-like noodles with a regular potato peeler and peel the zucchini lengthways. Set aside.

Using a carving knife, thinly slice the lamb or beef if it's not already sliced. Then place a medium-sized frying pan or skillet on high heat, sprinkle in the chives and add the meat, lightly browning on all sides. Using high heat will make the meat tender. If you have a good non-stick pan you won't need to use oil. Once the meat is cooked, remove from the heat and set aside while you heat the zucchini noodles. Use the same pan if you would like to combine the meat juices with the zucchini.

Place a medium-sized frying pan or wok over high heat. Add a dash of water (about 2 tablespoons) and once the water is simmering add the zucchini noodles (a few handfuls at a time) to lightly blanch for about 30 seconds. Once they are cooked, add these to serving bowls and continue cooking the remaining noodles until finished. Gently stir half the Cashew Cream or sauce of choice through the zucchini noodles. Then briefly heat the spring onions and red cabbage in the pan for a minute or less, so they remain crisp.

Top the zucchini noodles with the cabbage, spring onions and meat. Drizzle the remaining Cashew Cream on top for presentation.

Crispy Chicken

Serves 2, preparation time 20 minutes, cooking time 50 minutes

You are not missing out on a thing with this yummy baked chicken and mayo recipe — it's tasty and looks a wee bit naughty but it's so good for you, and your pretty pins will thank you later. Chickpea (besan, gram) flour is a gluten-free flour alternative that would work well too. If you are sensitive to amines remove the skin of the chicken before cooking. For a paleo meal, use no flour or try cassava flour and dried chives, and make Cashew Cream instead of the mayo (p. 142). If you are following Menu 4 follow the instructions for 'Quick Crispy Chicken' (opposite).

- ½ cup gluten-free plain/all purpose flour or oat flour (G), or no flour
- ¼ teaspoon quality sea salt
- 4–6 chicken drumsticks (depending on appetite and drumstick size)
- oil of choice (refer to 'Cooking oil options for your skin type', p. 92)
- ½ medium-sized leek
- 1 cup red cabbage
- 1 cup white cabbage
- 3 spring onions (shallots, scallions), roots removed
- Vegan Mayo (p. 146), to serve

Preheat the oven to 200°C (400°F) and line a baking tray with a silicon mat or baking (parchment) paper.

On a large plate combine the flour and salt, then coat each drumstick in a generous layer — this is optional as you can omit the flour and just use salt and dried chives, if preferred. Use your hands to press the flour into each drumstick so it is well coated.

Place a large non-stick frying pan or skillet on medium heat and add 1 tablespoon of oil (if you are not using flour you might not need oil, just make the pan hotter). Once the pan is hot, place the drumsticks into the pan to lightly brown. Using tongs, turn over after a few minutes and continue browning. Once the drumsticks are lightly browned, transfer them onto the baking tray and place them into the oven for 40 minutes or until crispy and cooked through.

Next, prepare the vegetables. Wash the leek to remove the dirt from the layers then finely slice, then finely shred the cabbages and spring onions. Five minutes before the chicken is ready, use the same frying pan you used for the chicken to cook the vegetables. Add a teaspoon of water and lightly sauté the leek and cabbage with the chicken juices for a couple of minutes, stirring occasionally. Add the spring onions, mix and turn off the heat.

Test if the chicken is cooked by pricking with a skewer to see if the juice runs clear, as the chicken must be cooked properly and not pink inside. Serve alongside the vegetables and top with a drizzle of Vegan Mayo.

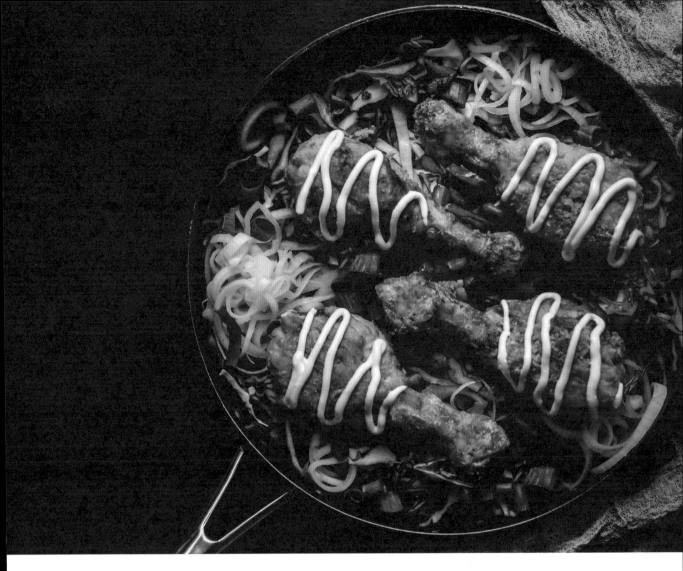

Variation: Quick Crispy Chicken

I love this delicious and simple recipe. Tips: the chicken must be skinless as there are amines in the skin, and ensure your meat is fresh from the butcher (only cook what you can eat today, as leftovers develop amines overnight). Don't make the mayo (sorry!) and use White Bean Sauce instead (p. 146).

Measurements are per person: thinly slice 1 skinless organic/free range chicken thigh fillet and sprinkle with ⅛–¼ teaspoon of quality sea salt and fresh chives. Preheat a non-stick frying pan or skillet on high heat and briefly cook each side of the chicken until golden and cooked through. Reduce heat to medium for the second side. Remove from heat and cook the vegetables as per the cooking instructions above.

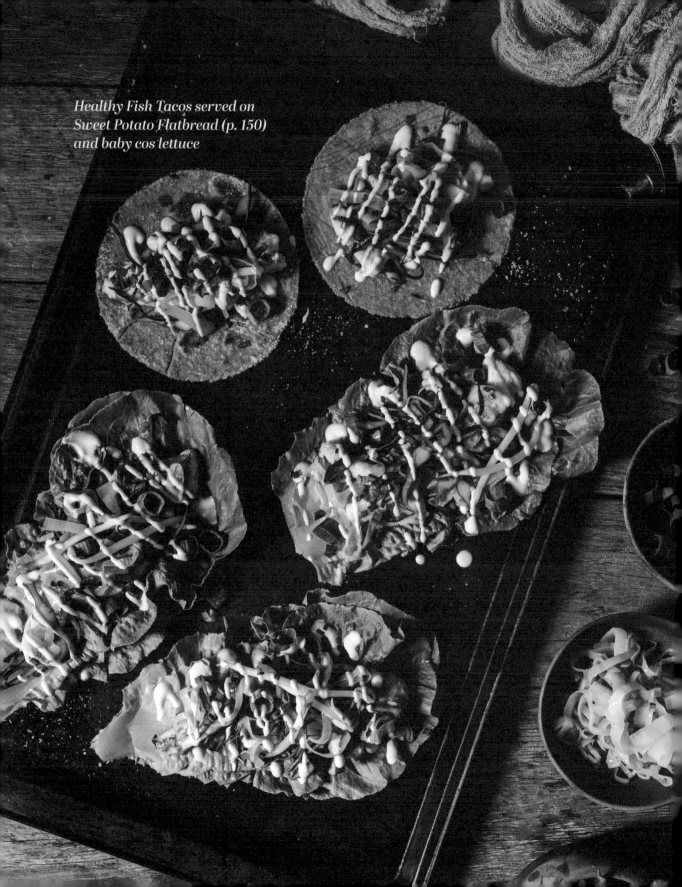

Healthy Fish Tacos served on Sweet Potato Flatbread (p. 150) and baby cos lettuce

Healthy Fish Tacos

Serves 2, preparation time 30 minutes, cooking time 10 minutes (if using lettuce leaf cups)

Serve these fabulous fish tacos in lettuce leaf cups, which is the quick gluten-free and paleo option, or if you have more time, make delicious Soft Tacos (p. 153). If you are following Menu 4 use iceberg lettuce (not cos/romaine) or make Oat and Leek Flatbread (p. 156) or Soft Tacos (p. 153); choose the freshest white fish (avoid the omega-3 rich fish list, and see 'The healthy fish list' on p. 94); avoid Cashew Cream and use no oil or a little sunflower oil or rice bran oil when cooking the fish.

- 1 iceberg lettuce or baby cos/romaine (S; fast/gluten-free option) or Oat and Leek Flatbread (p. 156) (G) or Soft Tacos (p. 153) (G)
- 300 g (10½ oz) flathead fillet or other small white fish of choice, skinned and deboned
- ⅛–¼ teaspoon quality sea salt (optional)
- ¼ cup washed and finely chopped fresh chives
- 1 teaspoon oil of choice (refer to 'Cooking oil options for your skin type', p. 92)
- ½ serve Caramelized Leek Sauce (p. 142)
- ½ cup washed and shredded red cabbage
- ¼ cup washed and finely sliced spring onions (shallots, scallions), washed
- ¼ cup bean sprouts or pea shoots/sprouts, washed (S) (optional; see p. 33)
- ½ serve Cashew Cream (optional, p. 142) (H)

Rinse the lettuce leaf cups (if using), gently shake them dry(ish) and place them onto serving bowls or plates. If using iceberg lettuce, you can use shallow condiment bowls to hold them upright.

Slice the fish into thin chunks about 2–3 cm (1–1½ in) in length and season lightly with salt and half of the chives. Place a non-stick frying pan or skillet on medium heat, add the oil and gently fry the fish on all sides until cooked through and slightly browned. You can lightly fry the cabbage and spring onion in the same pan or leave them raw, then mix them with the leek sauce.

Fill each wrap or lettuce leaf cup with the cabbage, leek sauce and spring onion mix, place the fish on top and sprinkle with sprouts (if using) and the remaining chives, and drizzle with Cashew Cream.

Chapter 14
Desserts

Banana Beet Nice Cream

Serves 3–4, preparation time 20 minutes (plus overnight freezing time)

The ice-cream alternative that will wow your taste buds … Beautifully coloured with the alkalizing goodness of beetroot and flavoured with sweet banana, which has mildly alkalizing properties thanks to the high level of potassium present. This recipe is lovely on its own or scoop it onto Oat Crepes (p. 195) or Banana Flour Pancakes (p. 195) for an amazing healthy dessert (or breakfast!).

- 4 medium bananas (A)
- 1 medium beetroot/beet, peeled (3 tablespoons /60 ml, when juiced) (S)
- 2 tablespoons plant-based milk of choice (p. 92)

Peel and chop the bananas, place them in an airtight container and freeze them overnight.

The next day, juice the beetroot in a juicer and, if needed, strain the juice to remove the pulp. If you do not have a juicer, grate the beetroot and blend it with ¼ cup of water in a high-speed blender and strain to remove the pulp.

In a food processor, combine 3 tablespoons (60 ml) of the beet juice with the frozen chopped bananas. If the machine won't blend the bananas, add a little plant-based milk 1 tablespoon at a time, and blend until smooth. Do not over-blend or add too much milk as this will make it too runny. Scrape the sides and blend again.

Nice cream can be served as is as a soft serve, or for a firmer dessert place it into the freezer for 30 minutes before serving. Freeze any leftovers. To soften leftovers that have frozen overnight, allow to partially thaw for about 30 minutes before serving.

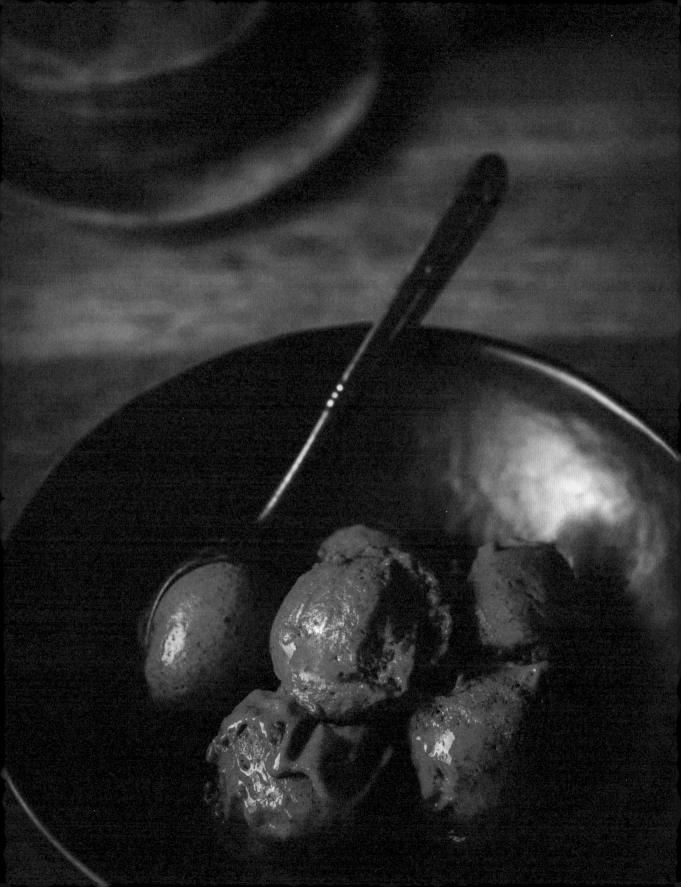

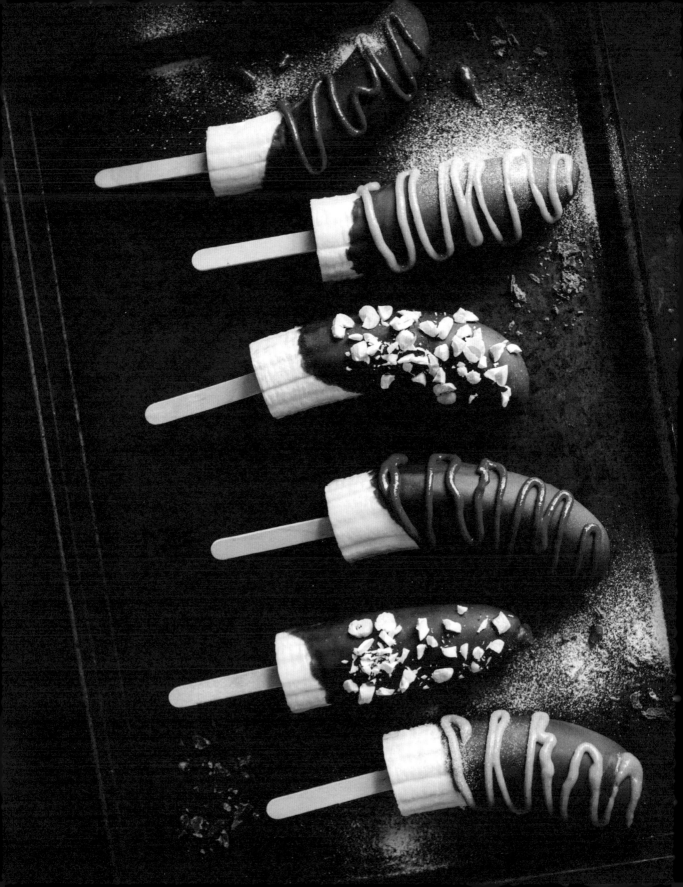

Banana Popsicles

Makes 10 popsicles, preparation time 30 minutes (plus 30 minutes freezing time)

Just looking at these popsicles can make you smile ... Bananas are a natural mood-booster, thanks to the tryptophan content which converts to serotonin — the feel-good neurotransmitter — and melatonin, which assists with sleep and relaxation. Keep them plain (the quick, easy option) or top them with crushed raw cashews, Beetroot Cashew Butter (p. 147) or Salted Caramel Nut Butter (p. 141). If you don't have popsicle sticks, make Banana Bites by coating frozen banana chunks in Carob Mylk Chocolate (p. 192) and set them on a lined tray in the freezer.

- 5 large ripe bananas, peeled and cut in half (A)
- 1 batch Carob Mylk Chocolate Bar mixture (p. 192; do not set in the refrigerator)
- 10 popsicle sticks (from a craft/art shop or large kitchen stores)

Before you begin, place the whole, unpeeled bananas into the freezer for 30 minutes so they are cold as the mylk chocolate will only set nicely (and quickly) when the bananas are cold — ensure you don't accidentally freeze them!

If you want to use the nut butter toppings make these now.

Prepare a plate or tray covered with baking (parchment) paper for your bananas and set aside.

Make the Carob Mylk Chocolate Bar mixture but do not put it in the refrigerator to set. Instead, place the mixture in a deep, narrow cup as this makes it easier to dip and coat the bananas in the melted chocolate.

Remove the bananas from the freezer, peel only the first one, cut it in half and insert a popsicle stick into each half. Holding the stick, dip the banana into the melted chocolate, rotating around to cover most of the banana. You might need to use one of your hands to lightly hold the base of the banana so it does not slide off the popsicle stick. If you are using toppings you can add the toppings to the first banana now (on one side only, and while the chocolate is still soft) as this will help the butters and nuts stick to the banana. You can use any method you wish for the nut butter application — we used a piping bag and a small round nozzle to create a thin zigzag design. Place the banana onto the tray to do this. If you are not using toppings, hold the choc-coated banana upright while the chocolate sets, then place it onto the lined tray.

Follow the same method with the other half of the banana then continue with the remaining bananas. If the chocolate mixture starts getting hard while you are still covering the bananas, place the container in some hot water to melt the mixture. Place the banana tray into the freezer and freeze overnight (serve them frozen). They will last about ten days in the freezer but if your family is like mine they probably won't last that long.

Carob Mylk Chocolate Bar

Makes 2 bars, preparation time 10 minutes, cooking time 10 minutes

There are two secrets to a good chocolate: first, make your sugar resemble icing sugar by blending it into a fine powder — this ensures a smoother chocolate feel in your mouth; and second, allow the melted chocolate to cool before you place it into the refrigerator, so the ingredients don't separate. You can use a high-speed blender or a stick blender.

A note about sugar: you could use any type of sugar as long as you blend it to resemble icing sugar, but maple sugar is the low salicylate/low amine option that is the best choice for people on Menu 3 or Menu 4. If you are following other menus or have healthy skin, feel free to substitute with another type of sugar if you can't find maple sugar. Do not use syrups such as maple syrup as the chocolate might curdle.

- 1 cup cacao butter buttons or shavings
- 2 tablespoons maple sugar
- ½ cup roasted carob powder (roasted works best as it's darker)

Optional toppings: rice bubbles/crispies (or plain puffed rice that has been toasted in a frying pan or skillet to make it crunchy), crushed raw cashews and a sprinkle of sea salt, or finely diced dried pear (preservative-free only). If you are following Menu 4 avoid using toppings.

Thin chocolate bars are easier to eat than one thick bar so use 2 x chocolate bar-shaped containers such as loaf tins (about 10 x 20 cm/ 4 x 8 in at the base). Line them with a large sheet of baking (parchment) paper, folded at the corners so the base and sides are covered and will cup the mixture without leaking. Alternatively, use moulds to make Easter Eggs or bite-sized chocolates (see Variation, below).

Use the double-boil method to protect the mixture from burning: fill a small saucepan with about 2 cm (1 in) of hot water and place a bowl on top, ensuring the bottom of the bowl does not touch the water. Place the cacao buttons in the bowl and gently heat on high heat until the buttons have melted. Remove the bowl from the heat and allow it to cool for about 10 minutes.

Meanwhile, make your sugar into fine icing sugar by placing it into a high-speed blender, blending on and off three times or until it resembles icing sugar. Strain it to remove any lumps and blend again if needed.

Then add the carob powder and melted cacao butter to the blender and blend until smooth (or use a stick blender and a high-sided/tall cup so you don't spatter yourself). Wait 5 minutes then blend it again. Once it has begun to thicken and cool, blend it again and quickly transfer the mixture to the loaf tins (sprinkle on the optional toppings now, if desired) and place the tins into the refrigerator to set; this will take a few hours. Once set, break the bars into decorative pieces or wedges, or alternatively you can leave the bar whole.

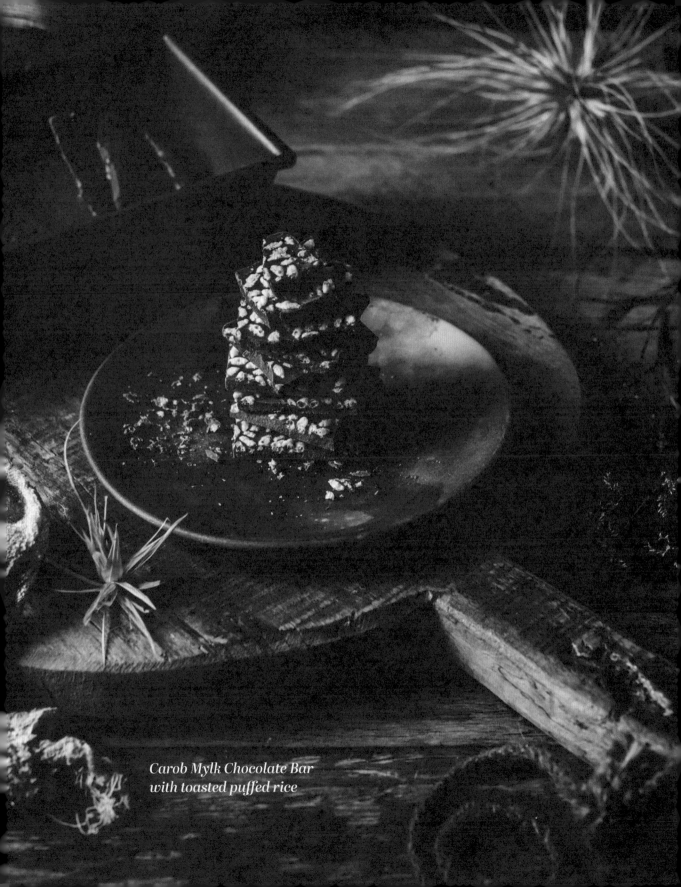

*Carob Mylk Chocolate Bar
with toasted puffed rice*

Banana Flour Pancakes
served with Banana
Beet Nice Cream (p. 188)

Banana Flour Pancakes

Makes 8+ pancakes or crepes, preparation time 5 minutes, cooking time 15 minutes

I love these served syrup-free, simply with pear and Cashew Butter (p. 141). For a special treat serve them with Banana Beet Nice Cream (p. 188). If you prefer paleo or gluten-free, make this recipe with green banana flour. I love the taste of green banana flour as it's sweeter than regular flour, but if you are new to it I suggest mixing ½ cup of green banana flour and ½ cup of oat flour, as it's a lovely prebiotic-rich combination with a milder flavour.

- 1 cup green banana flour (A) (or ½ cup green banana flour and ½ cup oat flour)
- ¼ cup tapioca flour/starch or arrowroot flour/starch
- 2½ cups cashew milk (H) or plant-based milk of choice (p. 92)

Toppings to choose from:
- Peeled pear (low salicylate/amine option)
- Banana slices (A)
- Papaya slices (A)
- Real maple syrup or rice malt/brown rice syrup (low salicylate option)
- Salted Caramel Nut Butter (p. 141) (H)

Combine the flours in a bowl, then add 1 cup of milk and mix vigorously until lump-free. Then gradually mix in the remaining 1½ cups of milk (using less milk initially helps to make the batter lump-free) until you have a smooth batter that is fairly thin for easy pouring.

Place a quality non-stick frying pan or skillet (a newer pan means you don't need to use oil) over medium heat, then measure out ¼ cup of batter and pour it into the pan. Lift the pan via the handle and, using a circular motion, spread the batter to make a thin pancake. Flip, and cook on both sides until lightly golden. Repeat until all the mixture is used. Serve with your toppings of choice.

Variation: Oat Crepes

Mix 1 cup of oat flour with ¼ cup of tapioca starch (or arrowroot starch) then gradually stir in 1¼ cups of oat milk until lump-free. Refer to the method above for cooking instructions. If the batter thickens and becomes hard to spread in the pan, add extra milk. Top with fresh sliced pear (and an optional drizzle of maple syrup, used sparingly).

gf   M4   pal   veg

Pink Pear Sorbet

Serves 4, preparation time 10 minutes (plus overnight freezing times)

This is such a lovely sorbet recipe that is so easy to make. It's so good for you too. If you have an ice-cream maker you can adapt this recipe by referring to the ice-cream maker instructions below. If you are following Menu 4, leave out the beetroot and guar gum.

- 4 large ripe pears
- 1 small–medium beetroot/beet (S) (you will need at least 3 tablespoons of juice)
- 1–3 tablespoons plant-based milk of choice (p. 92)
- ⅛ teaspoon guar gum (optional, for a smoother texture if using an ice-cream maker)

The night before, peel and chop the pears, place into a container with a lid and place in the freezer.

The next day, juice the beetroot in a juicing machine (or grate the beetroot and place ¼ cup of grated beetroot with ½ cup of water and blend in a high-speed blender), then strain the juice/water to remove the pulp.

Add the frozen pears and 2 tablespoons of beet juice to a regular food processor and process on low–medium speed. Stop and scrape down the sides, and if desired, add an extra 1–2 tablespoons of beet juice until the desired colour and consistency is achieved. Gradually add the

milk (too much will make it too runny so add 1 tablespoon at a time). Scrape down the sides and blend until smooth, but do not over-blend as it will melt. Serve immediately as a soft serve or place the sorbet into a container, seal with a lid and put it into the freezer for about 30 minutes to thicken. Freeze any leftovers. When serving leftovers, remove from the freezer, place onto the kitchen bench and allow to partially thaw for about 20–30 minutes to soften.

ICE-CREAM MAKER INSTRUCTIONS

Place the bowl of your ice-cream maker in the freezer for the time suggested on the instructions, then assemble the ice-cream maker. Blend the ingredients in a food processor and add at least 100 ml (3½ fl oz) of extra milk to the recipe and blend until smooth — ensure the mixture is runny, not chunky. Then pour the mixture through the shoot of the ice-cream maker. Mix until it has thickened; this may take about 10 minutes. Refer to the ice-cream maker instructions if necessary.

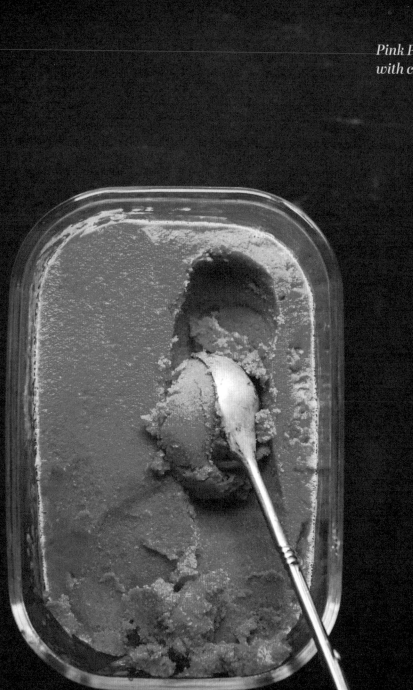

Pink Pear Sorbet made with creamy oat milk

Helpful resources

Here are some helpful resources to make your life easier ...

Healthy Skin Kitchen online program

If you need help while following my programs, my team of HSK (and Eczema Detox) trained nutritionists offer support, chat forums and step-by-step guidance for Food Intolerance Diagnosis (FID) and more, via my HSK online program.

How to get your kids loving vegies (and more)

Healthy Family, Happy Family: The complete healthy guide to feeding your family e-book from www.exislepublishing.com
Don't Tell Them It's Healthy online at healthyskinkitchen.com.

Shopping guides

If you wish to follow a low salicylate and low amine program, download one of the Eczema Diet Shopping Guides (at present there are shopping guides for the United States, Canada and Australia). See www.skinfriend.com and use the code DETOX101 for a free PDF copy, emailed to your inbox.

Food charts

Download a free histamine and salicylate food chart when you join my newsletter at www.skinfriend.com (scroll to the bottom of the website for the subscription box).

Skin Friend

www.skinfriend.com
Powder supplements: Skin Friend AM and Skin Friend PM
Skin care: 24-Hour Rescue Balm
Other: Oat and Zinc Bath Powder
Books: *The Eczema Detox* and *The Eczema Diet* by Karen Fischer
More products on the way ...

Synergie Skin

www.synergieskin.com
ÜberZinc (SPF15 face cream for all skin types), ReVeal, BAcne, Blem-X and Blemish Control Kit (for acne), Vitamin B (anti-ageing serum).

Online yoga and meditation

Essence of Living: www.essenceofliving.com.au
Honey Studio: www.kimberleybargenquast.com
Merrymaker Sisters (body positivity, great for teens): www.themerrymakersisters.com.

Recommended music

Spotify is a free app that houses all types of music and playlists (I recommend paying for a subscription if you love music). See www.spotify.com or search 'Spotify' on the app store on your smartphone; you can also download it onto your computer. I have created several wellness playlists for you. Search for these playlists by Skin Friend on Spotify (Skin Friend is my account name):

- » Vagus Nerve Wellness
- » Dance in the Kitchen (music while you cook)
- » Sleep Well.

Brain retraining

Dynamic Neural Retraining System (DNRS) by Annie Hopper: www.retrainingthebrain.com
The Gupta Program by Ashok Gupta: www.guptaprogram.com.

Recommended apps

Meditation: Meaning of Life Experiment (by Ashok Gupta)
Immunity training: Wim Hof Method
Music: Spotify

Chronic inflammatory response syndrome (CIRS)

Find a practitioner at www.survivingmold.com and do the online visual contrast test at www.survivingmold.com/store1/online-screening-test.

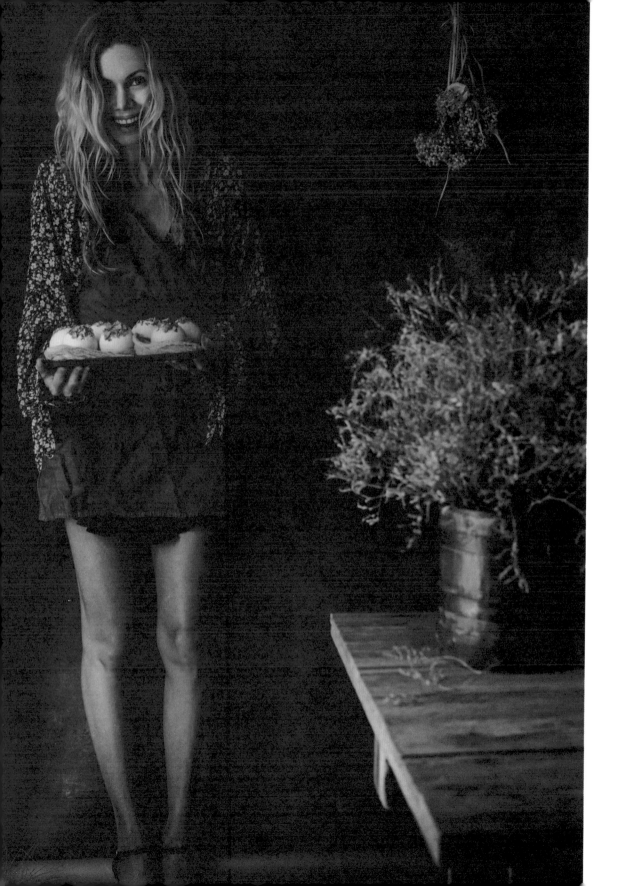

Gratitude

When I first became a nutritionist people said, 'How are you going to make any money?' I was told to go back into modelling or TV presenting. But I didn't want to. I just wanted to help people and write books. So thank you to the two people who have always believed in me: my parents. They are still amazed that I now cook and eat healthy food, as I was a typical unhealthy and lazy teenager. But with each career change I made, they never spoke their fears aloud — they trusted me even though they silently had doubts that their once shy and anxious daughter could talk on TV, be healthy and write books. My secret is a whole lot of self-belief and I'm sure that comes from my mother's can-do attitude.

I have many people to thank for their valuable input during the making of this book. My daughter Ayva and son Jack were my first recipe testers — thanks for your honesty (any recipe they did not love, did not make it into the book). Thank you to fellow nutritionist Katie Layland for your valuable assistance with the recipe development in this book — it has been wonderful working with you over the years at Skin Friend and Eczema Life.

Thank you Ayva Lily, Bonnie Taylor, Sarah Campbell, Kelly Macdonald and Grace Pettitt for your hand modelling and assistance in the photos and for your wonderful work at Skin Friend. And thank you to Gareth St John Thomas for publishing this book and editor/s Anouska Jones and Karen Gee for making my work better and to Mark Thacker for typesetting and making this book look beautiful. And a big thank you to my agent Selwa Anthony for having faith in me and thank you Tara Moss for introducing me to Selwa many years ago — this changed my life and made a lifelong goal to write books a reality.

I'm incredibly grateful to my online friends who made the ceramics that featured in the photos, including Anna-Marie from Made of Australia, Joy from Batch Ceramics and Sandra from All Fired Up Pottery. And a big virtual hug to photographers Anisa Sabet and Aimee Twigger for teaching me how to use my camera! A huge thank you to Charlie Rioux for your valuable help with our online Eczema Diet Support Group and the US and Canadian shopping guides.

My dad helped me to make the rustic timber desk (from 100-year-old fence palings from Bondi) which features heavily in the photos, so a special thank you for knowing how to make useful stuff. And thank you to Lyn McCreanor (www.inallthingsbeautiful.com), for taking the beautiful family photo on p. 7, which was taken in the Paddington Reservoir on Oatley Road (at the end of the street where I had my eczema clinic until 2018) — such great memories!

And a special hello to my former patients and readers who supplied feedback and testimonials over the years — thank you! You are the reason I keep writing books. And a special thank you to Kate Smith for sharing her journey with eczema at the beginning of this book — your email arrived a few days before I handed in this manuscript and I had to include your inspirational story. I was not able to include all of the other success stories sent to me, so I have added them to my website at www.eczemalife.com (thank you to everyone who supplied testimonials and before-and-after photos). Plus a special thank you to my cousins (Raelea, Grant, Lee, Maddy and Emma), Auntie Merle, Mum, Dad and my uncles for your feedback on my 'magic balms'. Thanks and hello to my sister Tracey — we love you and miss you. And a big thank you to Jeremy and Kirty Debray for the doors and kitchen props.

On another note, it was a difficult year for many of us due to the COVID-19 pandemic in 2020. So a special thanks to my yoga teachers including Michelle Cassidy, Kimberley Bargenquast, Hollie Bradley and Carla Papas who kept me fit and sane with your online classes, while I finished this book and during lockdown. Remember to enjoy life but also keep cooking for yourself because you create your body with your knife and fork, so it pays to know what you are eating.

A special thanks to Shad, Jacquee Saunders, Lou McGregor, Lorraine Gaffney, Shell Griffiths, Rachael Scobie, Katrina Warren, Megan Gale, Tali Jatali, Annie Bloom, Dominique Sutton, Katie Ashton, Tory Archbold, Lizzie Dart, Belinda Matheson, Libby-Jane Charleston, Jacinta Tynan, Lyn McPherson, Kirty Kruck, Anna Stokes, Jo Ferguson (I miss you beautiful) and all of my wonderful friends who helped me to feel connected and loved while on my own (via text and Zoom) during the pandemic. You kept me laughing while I finished this manuscript and it highlighted to me how important it is to stay connected with old friends and uplift others, so I dedicate this book to all of you.

Thank you for reading my book and for putting your trust in me. I wish you beautiful skin but most of all, remember to just love yourself more, eat while calm and be grateful for what you have, because you can feel good right now, wherever you are in your health and wellness journey.

Love, health and happiness,
Karen xx

Endnotes

Chapter 1

1. Rezzi, S., Ramadan, Z., Martin, F.P.J., Fay, L.B., Van Bladeren, P., Lindon, J.C., Nicholson, J.K. and Kochhar, S. 2007, 'Human metabolic phenotypes link directly to specific dietary preferences in healthy individuals', *Journal of Proteome Research*, 6 (11), pp. 4469–77; Alcock, J., Maley, C.C. and Aktipis, C.A. 2014, 'Is eating behavior manipulated by the gastrointestinal microbiota? Evolutionary pressures and potential mechanisms', *Bioessays*, 36 (10), pp. 940–49.
2. Alcock, J., Maley, C.C. and Aktipis, C.A. 2014.
3. Alcock, J., Maley, C.C. and Aktipis, C.A. 2014.
4. Fontana, L. and Partridge, L. 2015, 'Promoting health and longevity through diet: From model organisms to humans', *Cell*, 161 (1), pp. 106–18; Longo, V.D. and Mattson, M.P., 2014, 'Fasting: Molecular mechanisms and clinical applications', *Cell Metabolism*, 19 (2), pp.181–92.
5. Longo, V.D. 2014.
6. He, Y., Yin, J., Lei, J., Liu, F., Zheng, H., Wang, S., Wu, S., Sheng, H., McGovern, E. and Zhou, H. 2019, 'Fasting challenges human gut microbiome resilience and reduces Fusobacterium', *Medicine in Microecology*, p.100003.
7. Fontana, L. 2015; Longo, V.D. 2014.

Chapter 2

1. Solan, M. 2019, 'Ease anxiety and stress: Take a (belly) breather', Harvard Health Publishing, Harvard Medical School, retrieved from https://www.health.harvard.edu/blog/.
2. Breit, S., Kupferberg, A., Rogler, G. and Hasler, G. 2018, 'Vagus nerve as modulator of the brain–gut axis in psychiatric and inflammatory disorders', *Frontiers in Psychiatry*, 9, p. 44.
3. Breit, S. 2018; Bonaz, B., Sinniger, V. and Pellissier, S. 2016, 'Vagal tone: Effects on sensitivity, motility, and inflammation', *Neurogastroenterology and Motility*, 28 (4), pp. 455–62; Bonaz, B., Sinniger, V. and Pellissier, S. 2016, 'Anti inflammatory properties of the vagus nerve: Potential therapeutic implications of vagus nerve stimulation', *Journal of Physiology*, 594 (20), pp. 5781–90.
4. Gould, K. 2019, 'Vagus nerve: Your body's communication superhighway', *Live Science*, retrieved from www.livescience.com/vagus-nerve.
5. Porges, S.W. 1992, 'Vagal tone: A physiologic marker of stress vulnerability', *Pediatrics*, 90, pp. 498–504.
6. De Couck, M., Nijs, J. and Gidron, Y. 2014, 'You may need a nerve to treat pain: The neurobiological rationale for vagal nerve activation in pain management', *Clinical Journal of Pain*, 30 (12), pp. 1099–1105.
7. Lin, T.K., Zhong, L. and Santiago, J.L. 2017, 'Association between stress and the HPA axis in the atopic dermatitis', *International Journal of Molecular Sciences*, 18 (10), p. 2131.
8. Choe, S.J., et.al. 2018, 'Psychological stress deteriorates skin barrier function by activating 11 -hydroxysteroid dehydrogenase 1 and the HPA axis', *Scientific Reports*, 8 (1), pp. 1–11.
9. Chan, C.W., et.al. 2018, 'The association between maternal stress and childhood eczema: A systematic review', *International Journal of Environmental Research and Public Health*, 15 (3), p. 395.
10. Lin, T.K. 2017.
11. Bonaz, B., Sinniger, V. and Pellissier, S. 2017, 'The vagus nerve in the neuro-immune axis: Implications in the pathology of the gastrointestinal tract', *Frontiers in Immunology*, 8, p. 1452.
12. Bonaz, B., Sinniger, V. and Pellissier, S. 2016.
13. Field, T. and Diego, M. 2008, 'Vagal activity, early growth and emotional development', *Infant Behavior and Development*, 31 (3), pp. 361–73; McLaughlin, K.A., Rith-Najarian, L., Dirks, M.A. and Sheridan, M.A. 2015, 'Low vagal tone magnifies the association between psychosocial stress exposure and internalizing psychopathology in adolescents', *Journal of Clinical Child & Adolescent Psychology*, 44 (2), pp. 314–28.
14. Porter, F.L., Porges, S.W. and Marshall, R.E. 1988, 'Newborn pain cries and vagal tone: Parallel changes in response to circumcision', *Child Development*, pp. 495–505.
15. McLaughlin, K.A. et al. 2015.
16. Kirchner, A., Stefan, H., Schmelz, M., Haslbeck, K.M. and Birklein, F. 2002, 'Influence of vagus nerve stimulation on histamine-induced itching', *Neurology*, 59 (1), pp. 108–112.
17. Tran, B.W., Papoiu, A.D., Russoniello, C.V., Wang, H., Patel, T.S., Chan, Y.H. and Yosipovitch, G. 2010, 'Effect of itch, scratching and mental stress on autonomic nervous system function in atopic dermatitis', *Acta Dermato-venereologica*, 90 (4), pp. 354–61.
18. Bosmans, G., Appeltans, I., Stakenborg, N., Gomez Pinilla, P.J., Florens, M.V., Aguilera Lizarraga, J., Matteoli, G. and Boeckxstaens, G.E. 2019, 'Vagus nerve stimulation dampens intestinal inflammation in a murine model of experimental food allergy', *Allergy*, 74 (9), pp. 1748–59.
19. Bonaz, B., Bazin, T. and Pellissier, S. 2018, 'The vagus nerve at the interface of the microbiota-gut-brain axis', *Frontiers in Neuroscience*, 12, p. 49.

20. Bonaz, B., Bazin, T. and Pellissier, S. 2018.
21. McLaughlin, K.A. et al. 2015.
22. Sack, M., Hopper, J.W. and Lamprecht, F. 2004, 'Low respiratory sinus arrhythmia and prolonged psychophysiological arousal in posttraumatic stress disorder: Heart rate dynamics and individual differences in arousal regulation', *Biological Psychiatry*, 55 (3), pp. 284–90.
23. McLaughlin, K.A. et al. 2015.
24. McLaughlin, K.A. et al. 2015.
25. Park, G. and Thayer, J.F. 2014, 'From the heart to the mind: Cardiac vagal tone modulates top-down and bottom-up visual perception and attention to emotional stimuli', *Frontiers in Psychology*, 5, p. 278; Lyonfields, J.D., Borkovec, T.D. and Thayer, J.F. 1995, 'Vagal tone in generalized anxiety disorder and the effects of aversive imagery and worrisome thinking', *Behavior Therapy*, 26 (3), pp. 457–66.
26. Park, G. and Thayer, J.F. 2014.
27. Park, G. and Thayer, J.F. 2014.
28. Park, G. and Thayer, J.F. 2014.
29. Jones, R.M., Buhr, A.P., Conture, E.G., Tumanova, V., Walden, T.A. and Porges, S.W. 2014, 'Autonomic nervous system activity of preschool-age children who stutter', *Journal of Fluency Disorders*, 41, pp. 12–31; Doruk, A., Tuerkbay, T., Yelboga, Z., Ciyiltepe, M., Iyisoy, A., Suetcigil, L. and Öz ahin, A. 2008, 'Autonomic nervous system imbalance in young adults with developmental stuttering', *Klinik Psikofarmakoloji Bulteni*, 18 (4).
30. Diamond, A., Kenney, C. and Jankovic, J. 2006, 'Effect of vagal nerve stimulation in a case of Tourette's syndrome and complex partial epilepsy', *Movement Disorders: Official journal of the Movement Disorder Society*, 21 (8), pp. 1273–5; Hawksley, J., Cavanna, A.E. and Nagai, Y. 2015, 'The role of the autonomic nervous system in Tourette syndrome', *Frontiers in Neuroscience*, 9, p. 117.
31. Diamond, A., Kenney, C. and Jankovic, J. 2006.
32. Ulloa, L. 2005, 'The vagus nerve and the nicotinic anti-inflammatory pathway', *Nature Reviews Drug Discovery*, 4 (8), pp. 673–84; Taylor, L., Loerbroks, A., Herr, R.M., Lane, R.D., Fischer, J.E. and Thayer, J.F. 2011, 'Depression and smoking: mediating role of vagal tone and inflammation', *Annals of Behavioral Medicine*, 42 (3), pp. 334–40.
33. Abrahamsson, T.R., et.al. 2011, 'A Th1/Th2 associated chemokine imbalance during infancy in children developing eczema, wheeze and sensitization', *Clinical & Experimental Allergy*, 41 (12), pp. 1729–39.
34. Bosmans, G. et al. 2019.
35. Bosmans, G. et al. 2019.
36. Solan, M. 2019.
37. Ditto, B., Eclache, M. and Goldman, N. 2006, 'Short-term autonomic and cardiovascular effects of mindfulness body scan meditation', *Annals of Behavioral Medicine*, 32 (3), pp. 227–34.
38. Sarang, P. and Telles, S. 2006, 'Effects of two yoga based relaxation techniques on heart rate variability (HRV)', *International Journal of Stress Management*, 13 (4), p. 460.
39. Peachman, R.R. 2017, 'Electrical grounding technique may improve health outcomes of NICU babies', *Penn State News*, retrieved from https://www.psu.edu/.
40. DiSalvo, D. 2009, 'Forget survival of the fittest: It is kindness that counts', *Scientific American: Mind*, retrieved from www.scientificamerican.com/article/forget-survival-of-the-fittest.
41. DiSalvo, D. 2009.
42. DiSalvo, D. 2009.
43. Hamilton, D.R. 2014, 'Does your brain distinguish real from imaginary?' retrieved from https://drdavidhamilton.com/does-your-brain-distinguish-real-from-imaginary.
44. Hamilton, D.R. 2014.
45. Kok, B.E., Coffey, K.A., Cohn, M.A., Catalino, L.I., Vacharkulksemsuk, T., Algoe, S.B., Brantley, M. and Fredrickson, B.L. 2013, 'How positive emotions build physical health: Perceived positive social connections account for the upward spiral between positive emotions and vagal tone', *Psychological Science*, 24 (7), pp. 1123–32.
46. Korb, A. 2012, 'The grateful brain', *Psychology Today*, retrieved from www.psychologytoday.com/au
47. Porges, S.W. 1992.

Chapter 3
1. Glatz, Z., Kovar, J., Macholan, L. and Pec, P. 1987, 'Pea *(Pisum sativum)* diamine oxidase contains pyrroloquinoline quinone as a cofactor', *Biochemical journal*, 242 (2), p. 603.
2. Boehm, T., et.al. 2019, 'Massive release of the histamine degrading enzyme diamine oxidase during severe anaphylaxis in mastocytosis patients', *Allergy*, 74 (3), pp. 583–93.
3. Huizen, J. 2018, 'Which foods are high in histamine?' *Medical News Today*, retrieved from https://www.medicalnewstoday.com/.
4. Huizen, J. 2018.
5. Ionescu, G. and Kiehl, R. 1989, 'Cofactor levels of mono- and diamine oxidase in atopic eczema', *Allergy*, 44, pp. 298–300.
6. Masini, E., Bani, D., Marzocca, C., Mateescu, M.A., Mannaioni, P.F., Federico, R. and Mondovì, B. 2007, 'Pea seedling histaminase as a novel therapeutic approach to anaphylactic and inflammatory disorders', *Scientific World Journal*, 7, pp. 888–902.
7. Joneja, J.M. 2014, 'Diamine oxidase from pea seedlings, *Allergy Nutrition*, retrieved from www.allergynutrition.com; Glatz, Z. 1987.
8. Joneja, J.M. 2014.
9. Karim, A., Wahab, A.W., Raya, I., Natsir, H. and Arif, A.R. 2018, 'Utilization of diamine oxidase enzyme from mung bean sprouts

(*Vigna radiata L*) for histamine biosensors', *Journal of Physics: Conference Series*, vol. 979, no. 1, p. 012014.

10. Hussain, E.A., Sadiq, Z. and Zia-Ul-Haq, M. 2018, 'Role of betalain in human health', in *Betalains: Biomolecular aspects* (pp. 97–107); Clifford, T., Howatson, G., West, D.J. and Stevenson, E.J. 2015, 'The potential benefits of red beetroot supplementation in health and disease', *Nutrients*, 7 (4), pp. 2801–22.

11. Yi, M.R., Kang, C.H. and Bu, H.J. 2017, 'Antioxidant and anti-inflammatory activity of extracts from red beet (*Beta vulagaris*) root', *Korean Journal of Food Preservation*, 24 (3), pp. 413–20; Clifford, T. 2015.

12. Akond, A.S.M.G.M., et.al. 2011, 'Anthocyanin, total polyphenols and antioxidant activity of common bean', *American Journal of Food Technology*, 6 (5), pp. 385–94; William Reed Business Media 2003, 'Black beans high in antioxidant ratings', retrieved from https://www.nutraingredients.com.

13. Goyal, A., Sharma, V., Upadhyay, N., Gill, S. and Sihag, M. 2014, 'Flax and flaxseed oil: An ancient medicine and modern functional food', *Journal of Food Science and Technology*, 51 (9), pp. 1633–53.

14. Goyal, A. et al. 2014.

15. Leizer, C., Ribnicky, D., Poulev, A., Dushenkov, S. and Raskin, I. 2000, 'The composition of hemp seed oil and its potential as an important source of nutrition', *Journal of Nutraceuticals, Functional & Medical Foods*, 2 (4), pp. 35–53.

16. Callaway, J., et.al., 2005. Efficacy of dietary hempseed oil in patients with atopic dermatitis. *Journal of Dermatological Treatment*, 16 (2), pp. 87–94.

17. Fattorusso, E., Lanzotti, V., Taglialatela-Scafati, O. and Cicala, C. 2001, 'The flavonoids of leek, *Allium porrum*', *Phytochemistry*, 57 (4), pp. 565–9; Kim, K., Kim, S., Moh, S.H. and Kang, H. 2015, 'Kaempferol inhibits vascular smooth muscle cell migration by modulating BMP-mediated miR-21 expression', *Molecular and Cellular Biochemistry*, 407 (1–2), pp. 143–9; Calderon-Montano, J.M., Burgos-Morón, E., Pérez-Guerrero, C. and López-Lázaro, M. 2011, 'A review on the dietary flavonoid kaempferol', *Mini Reviews in Medicinal Chemistry*, 11 (4), pp. 298–344.

18. Roberfroid, M.B. 2005, 'Introducing inulin-type fructans', *British Journal of Nutrition*, 93 (S1), pp. S13–25.

19. Daou, C. and Zhang, H. 2012, 'Oat beta glucan: Its role in health promotion and prevention of diseases', *Comprehensive Reviews in Food Science and Food Safety*, 11 (4), pp. 355–65.

20. Daou, C. and Zhang, H. 2012.

21. Daou, C. and Zhang, H. 2012.

22. Kahlon, T.S. and Smith, G.E. 2007, 'In vitro binding of bile acids by bananas, peaches, pineapple, grapes, pears, apricots and nectarines', *Food Chemistry*, 101 (3), pp. 1046–51.

23. Wedick, N.M., et.al., 2012. Dietary flavonoid intakes and risk of type 2 diabetes in US men and women. *The American Journal of Clinical Nutrition*, 95(4), pp. 925-933.

24. Ash, M. 2013, 'Clinical pearls: Papaya as a foundation for gut health', *Clinical Education*, retrieved from clinicaleducation.org.

25. Parvu, A.E., Parvu, M., Vlase, L., Miclea, P., Mot, A.C. and Silaghi-Dumitrescu, R. 2014, 'Anti-inflammatory effects of *Allium schoenoprasum* L. leaves', *J Physiol Pharmacol*, 65 (2), pp. 309–15.

26. Wiedermann, et.al. 1996, 'Vitamin A deficiency increases inflammatory responses', *Scandinavian Journal of Immunology*, 44 (6), pp. 578–84; Hunt, T.K. 1986, 'Vitamin A and wound healing', *Journal of the American Academy of Dermatology*, 15 (4), pp. 817–21.

27. Paliwal, S., Sundaram, J. and Mitragotri, S. 2005, 'Induction of cancer-specific cytotoxicity towards human prostate and skin cells using quercetin and ultrasound', *British Journal of Cancer*, 92 (3), pp. 499–502.

28. Ju, R., Zheng, S., Luo, H., Wang, C., Duan, L., Sheng, Y., Zhao, C., Xu, W. and Huang, K. 2017, 'Purple sweet potato attenuate weight gain in high fat diet induced obese mice', *Journal of Food Science*, 82 (3), pp. 787–93.

29. Ju, R. et al. 2017.

30. Nijhoff, W.A., et.al. 1995, 'Effects of consumption of Brussels sprouts on intestinal and lymphocytic glutathione S-transferases in humans', *Carcinogenesis*, 16 (9), pp. 2125–8.

31. Li, F., Hullar, M.A., Schwarz, Y. and Lampe, J.W. 2009, 'Human gut bacterial communities are altered by addition of cruciferous vegetables to a controlled fruit-and-vegetable-free diet', *Journal of Nutrition*, 139 (9), pp. 1685–91; Nijhoff, W.A., et.al., 1995; Kunimasa, K., Kobayashi, T., Kaji, K. and Ohta, T. 2010, 'Antiangiogenic effects of indole-3-carbinol and 3, 3'-diindolylmethane are associated with their differential regulation of ERK1/2 and Akt in tube-forming HUVEC', *Journal of Nutrition*, 140 (1), pp. 1–6.

32. Kahlon, T.S., Chapman, M.H. and Smith, G.E. 2007, 'In vitro binding of bile acids by spinach, kale, brussels sprouts, broccoli, mustard greens, green bell pepper, cabbage and collards', *Food Chemistry*, 100 (4), pp. 1531–6.

33. Harshman, S.G. and Shea, M.K. 2016, 'The role of vitamin K in chronic aging diseases: Inflammation, cardiovascular disease, and osteoarthritis', *Current Nutrition Reports*, 5 (2), pp. 90–98.

34. Kahlon, T.S., Chiu, M.C.M. and Chapman, M.H. 2008, 'Steam cooking significantly improves in vitro bile acid binding of collard greens, kale, mustard greens,

broccoli, green bell pepper, and cabbage', *Nutrition Research*, 28 (6), pp. 351–7.

35. Mitsou, E.K., Kougia, E., Nomikos, T., Yannakoulia, M., Mountzouris, K.C. and Kyriacou, A. 2011, 'Effect of banana consumption on faecal microbiota: A randomised, controlled trial', *Anaerobe*, 17 (6), pp. 384–7.

36. Bezerra, C.V., Rodrigues, A.M.D.C., Amante, E.R. and Silva, L.H.M.D. 2013, 'Nutritional potential of green banana flour obtained by drying in spouted bed', *Revista Brasileira de Fruticultura*, 35 (4), pp. 1140–46; Higgins, J.A. 2004, 'Resistant starch: Metabolic effects and potential health benefits'. *Journal of AOAC International*, 87 (3), pp. 761–8.

37. Karababa, E. and Coskuner, Y. 2013, 'Physical properties of carob bean (*Ceratonia siliqua L.*): An industrial gum yielding crop', *Industrial Crops and Products*, 42, pp. 440–46.

38. Murray, M.T. and Pizzorno J. 2010, *The Encyclopedia of Healing Foods*, Simon & Schuster, New York.

39. Murray, M.T. and Pizzorno J. 2010.

40. Murray, M.T. and Pizzorno J. 2010.

41. Murray, M.T. and Pizzorno J. 2010; Musa Özcan, M., Arslan, D. and Gökçalik, H. 2007, 'Some compositional properties and mineral contents of carob (*Ceratonia siliqua*) fruit, flour and syrup', *International Journal of Food Sciences and Nutrition*, 58 (8), pp. 652–8.

42. Gruendel, S., et.al. 2006, 'Carob pulp preparation rich in insoluble dietary fiber and polyphenols enhances lipid oxidation and lowers postprandial acylated ghrelin in humans', *Journal of Nutrition*, 136 (6), pp. 1533–8.

43. Kimata, H. 2007, 'Viewing humorous film improves night-time wakening in children with atopic dermatitis', *Indian pediatrics*, 44 (4), p.281.

44. Kimata, H. 2007.

45. Hagiwara, A., et.al. 2002, 'Prevention by natural food anthocyanins, purple sweet potato color and red cabbage color, of 2-amino-1-methyl-6-phenylimidazo [4, 5-B] pyridine (phip)-associated colorectal carcinogenesis in rats', *Journal of Toxicological Sciences*, 27 (1), pp. 57–68; Charron, C.S., Clevidence, B.A., Britz, S.J. and Novotny, J.A. 2007, 'Effect of dose size on bioavailability of acylated and nonacylated anthocyanins from red cabbage (*Brassica oleracea L.* Var. *capitata*)', *Journal of Agricultural and Food Chemistry*, 55 (13), pp. 5354–62.

46. Oancea, S. and Oprean, L. 2011, 'Anthocyanins, from biosynthesis in plants to human health benefits', *Acta Universitatis Cinbinesis, Series E: Food Technology*, 15(1).

47. Singh, J., et.al. 2006, 'Antioxidant phytochemicals in cabbage (*Brassica oleracea L.* var. *capitata*)', *Scientia Horticulturae*, 108 (3), pp. 233–7; Enye, J.C., et.al. 2013, 'Evaluation of the healing effects of aqueous extracts of *Musa Paradisiaca* (unripe plantain) and *Brassica oleracea* (cabbage) on peptic ulcer', *IOSR J Dental Med Sci*, 8, pp. 40–46.

48. Enye, J.C., et.al. 2013.

49. Kataria, K., Srivastava, A. and Dhar, A. 2013, 'Management of lactational mastitis and breast abscesses: Review of current knowledge and practice', *Indian Journal of Surgery*, 75 (6), pp. 430–35.

Chapter 4

1. Hodges, R.E. et al. 1969, 'Experimental scurvy in man', *American Journal of Clinical Nutrition*, vol. 22 (5), pp 535–48.

2. Velandia, B., Centor, R.M., McConnell, V. and Shah, M. 2008, 'Scurvy is still present in developed countries', *Journal of General Internal Medicine*, 23 (8), p. 1281; Wang, A.H. and Still, C. 2007, 'Old world meets modern: A case report of scurvy', *Nutrition in Clinical Practice*, 22 (4), pp. 445–8; Holley, A.D., Osland, E., Barnes, J., Krishnan, A. and Fraser, J.F. 2011, 'Scurvy: Historically a plague of the sailor that remains a consideration in the modern intensive care unit', *Internal Medicine Journal*, 41 (3), pp. 283–5; Wijkmans, R.A. and Talsma, K. 2016, 'Modern scurvy', *Journal of Surgical Case Reports*, (1), p. rjv168.

3. Brown, M.J. and Beier, K. 2018, 'Vitamin B6 deficiency (Pyridoxine)', in *StatPearls [Internet]*, StatPearls Publishing; Vilter, R.W., Mueller, J.F., Glazer, H.S., Jarrold, T., Abraham, J., Thompson, C. and Hawkins, V.R. 1953, 'The effect of vitamin B6 deficiency induced by desoxypyridoxine in human beings', *Journal of laboratory and clinical medicine*, 42 (3), pp. 335–57; Gilson, R.C., Wallis, L., Yeh, J. and Gilson, R.T. 2018, 'Dementia, diarrhea, desquamating shellac-like dermatitis revealing late-onset cobalamin C deficiency', *JAAD case reports*, 4 (1), p. 91.

4. Cabrini, L., et.al. 1998, 'Vitamin B6 deficiency affects antioxidant defences in rat liver and heart', *IUBMB Life*, 46 (4), pp. 689–97.

5. Piraccini, B.M., Berardesca, E., Fabbrocini, G., Micali, G. and Tosti, A. 2019, 'Biotin: overview of the treatment of diseases of cutaneous appendages and of hyperseborrhea', *Giornale italiano di dermatologia e venereologia: organo ufficiale, Societa italiana di dermatologia e sifilografia*, 154 (5), pp. 557–66; Lipner, S.R. and Scher, R.K. 2018, 'Biotin for the treatment of nail disease: What is the evidence?' *Journal of Dermatological Treatment*, 29 (4), pp. 411–14.

6. Sydenstricker, V.P., Singal, S.A., Briggs, A.P., DeVaughn, N.M. and Isbell, H. 1942, 'Observations on the egg white injury in man: And its cure with a biotin

concentrate', *Journal of the American Medical Association*, 118 (14), pp. 1199–1200; Gilson, R.C., Wallis, L., Yeh, J. and Gilson, R.T. 2018; Lipner, S.R. and Scher, R.K. 2018.

7. Trüeb, R.M. 2016, 'Serum biotin levels in women complaining of hair loss', *International Journal of Trichology*, 8 (2), p. 73.

8. Lipner, S.R. and Scher, R.K. 2018.

9. Sydenstricker, V.P. et al. 1942.

10. Gupta, M., Mahajan, V.K., Mehta, K.S. and Chauhan, P.S. 2014, 'Zinc therapy in dermatology: a review', *Dermatology research and practice*, 2014.

11. Cordain, L., Lindeberg, S., Hurtado, M., Hill, K., Eaton, S.B. and Brand-Miller, J. 2002, 'Acne vulgaris: A disease of Western civilization', *Archives of Dermatology*, 138 (12), pp. 1584–90.

12. Foster, R. 2019, 'Zinc deficiency and the skin', *Australasian College of Dermatologists*, retrieved from www.dermcoll.edu.au/atoz/zinc-deficiency-skin.

13. Gupta, M.et al. 2014; Foster, R. 2019.

14. Gupta, M. et al. 2014; Foster, R. 2019.

15. Dreno, B., Amblard, P., Agache, P., Sirot, S. and Litoux, P. 1989, 'Low doses of zinc gluconate for inflammatory acne', *Acta dermato-venereologica*, 69 (6), pp. 541–3; Gupta, M. et al. 2014.

16. Gupta, M. et al. 2014.

17. Gupta, M. et al. 2014.

18. Ozuguz, P., et.al. 2014, 'Evaluation of serum vitamins A and E and zinc levels according to the severity of acne vulgaris', *Cutaneous and Ocular Toxicology*, 33 (2), pp. 99–102.

19. Al Alawi, A.M., Majoni, S.W. and Falhammar, H. 2018, 'Magnesium and human health: Perspectives and research directions', *International Journal of Endocrinology*.

20. Al Alawi, A.M., Majoni, S.W. and Falhammar, H. 2018; Hruby, A., et.al. 2014, 'Magnesium intake is inversely associated with coronary artery calcification: The Framingham Heart Study', *JACC: Cardiovascular Imaging*, 7 (1), pp. 59–69.

21. Al Alawi, A.M., Majoni, S.W. and Falhammar, H., 2018; Najafi, M., Hamidian, R., Haghighat, B., Fallah, N., Tafti, H.A., Karimi, A. and Boroumand, M.A. 2007, 'Magnesium infusion and postoperative atrial fibrillation: A randomized clinical trial', *Acta Anaesthesiologica Sinica*, 45 (2), p. 89.

22. Al Alawi, A.M. et al. 2018.

23. Boyle, N., Lawton, C. and Dye, L. 2017, 'The effects of magnesium supplementation on subjective anxiety and stress — a systematic review', *Nutrients*, 9 (5), p. 429.

24. Lee, S.H., Jeong, S.K. and Ahn, S.K. 2006, 'An update of the defensive barrier function of skin', *Yonsei Medical Journal*, 47 (3), pp. 293–306.

25. Rinnerthaler, M. and Richter, K. 2018, 'The influence of calcium on the skin pH and epidermal barrier during aging', *pH of the Skin: Issues and Challenges*, 54, pp. 79–86.

26. Lee, S.H. et al. 2006.

27. Arul, S., Dayalan, H., Jegadeesan, M. and Damodharan, P. 2016, 'Induction of differentiation in psoriatic keratinocytes by propylthiouracil and fructose', *BBA Clinical*, 6, pp. 82–6.

28. Willett, W.C. and Ludwig, D.S. 2020, 'Milk and health', *New England Journal of Medicine*, 382 (7), pp. 644–54.

29. Bannai, M. and Kawai, N. 2012, 'New therapeutic strategy for amino acid medicine: Glycine improves the quality of sleep', *Journal of Pharmacological Sciences*, 118 (2), pp. 145–8.

30. Karthikeyan, K. and Thappa, D.M. 2002, 'Pellagra and skin', *International Journal of Dermatology*, 41 (8), pp. 476–81.

31. Wang, W. and Liang, B. 2012, 'Case report of mental disorder induced by niacin deficiency', *Shanghai Archives of Psychiatry*, 24 (6), p. 352.

32. Karthikeyan, K. and Thappa, D.M. 2002.

33. Wang, W. and Liang, B. 2012,

34. Kamanna, V.S., Ganji, S.H. and Kashyap, M.L. 2009, 'The mechanism and mitigation of niacin induced flushing', *International Journal of Clinical Practice*, 63 (9), pp. 1369–77.

35. De Spirt, S. et al. 2009, 'Intervention with flaxseed and borage oil supplements modulates skin condition in women', *British Journal of Nutrition*, 101, pp. 440–45.

36. Storey, A., et.al. 2005, 'Eicosapentaenoic acid and docosahexaenoic acid reduce UVB- and TNF-a-induced IL-8 secretion in keratinocytes and UVB-induced IL-8 in fibroblasts', *Journal of Investigative Dermatology*, 124 (1), pp. 248–55; Sierra, S., et.al. 2008, 'Dietary eicosapentaenoic acid and docosahexaenoic acid equally incorporate as decosahexaenoic acid in different inflammatory effects', *Nutrition*, 24 (3), pp. 245–54.

37. Papaioannou, R. and Pfeiffer, C.C. 1984, 'Sulfite sensitivity-unrecognized threat: Is molybdenum deficiency the cause?' *Journal of Orthomolecular Psychiatry*, 13 (2), pp. 105–10.

38. Abumrad, N.N. 1984, 'Molybdenum — is it an essential trace metal?' *Bulletin of the New York Academy of Medicine*, 60 (2), p. 163.

39. Richie, J.P., Nichenametla, S., Neidig, W., Calcagnotto, A., Haley, J.S., Schell, T.D. and Muscat, J.E. 2015, 'Randomized controlled trial of oral glutathione supplementation on body stores of glutathione', *European Journal of Nutrition*, 54 (2), pp. 251–63.

40. Richie, J.P., et.al. 2015.

Part 2

Chapter 5

1. Sur, R., Nigam, A., Grote, D., Liebel, F. and Southall, M.D. 2008, 'Avenanthramides, polyphenols from oats, exhibit anti-inflammatory and anti-itch activity', *Archives of Dermatological Research*, 300 (10), p. 569.
2. Sur, R. et al. 2008.
3. Zeng, W. and Endo, Y. 2019, 'Lipid characteristics of camellia seed oil', *Journal of Oleo Science*, p.ess18234; Kim, S.K. and Karadeniz, F. 2012, 'Biological importance and applications of squalene and squalane', *Advances in Food and Nutrition Research*, 65, pp. 223–33.
4. Honfo, F.G., Akissoe, N., Linnemann, A.R., Soumanou, M. and Van Boekel, M.A. 2014, 'Nutritional composition of shea products and chemical properties of shea butter: A review', *Critical Reviews in Food Science and Nutrition*, 54 (5), pp. 673–86.
5. Chawla, K.K., Bencharitiwong, R., Ayuso, R., Grishina, G. and Nowak-Wegrzyn, A. 2011, 'Shea butter contains no IgE-binding soluble proteins', *Journal of Allergy and Clinical Immunology*, 127 (3), p. 680; 'Shea nuts', 2019, Anaphylaxis Campaign, peer-reviewed article, retrieved from https://www.anaphylaxis.org.uk.
6. Drake, D. 1997, 'Antibacterial activity of baking soda', *Compendium of Continuing Education in Dentistry*, (Jamesburg, NJ: 1995). Supplement, 18 (21), pp. S17–21.
7. Verdolini, R., et.al. 2005, 'Old fashioned sodium bicarbonate baths for the treatment of psoriasis in the era of futuristic biologics: An old ally to be rescued', *Journal of Dermatological Treatment*, 16 (1), pp. 26–9.
8. Yousef, J.M. and Danial, E.N. 2012, 'In vitro antibacterial activity and minimum inhibitory concentration of zinc oxide and nano-particle zinc oxide against pathogenic strains', *Journal of Health Sciences*, 2 (4), pp. 38–42.

Chapter 6

1. Gilson, R.C. et al. 2018.
2. Campos, M., 2017, 'Leaky gut: What is it, and what does it mean for you?', *Harvard Heath Publishing*, Harvard Medical School, retrieved from https://www.health.harvard.edu/blog/.
3. Rapaport, M. 'What is red skin syndrome?' *Understanding Red Skin Syndrome*, retrieved from www.red-skin-syndrome.com.

Chapter 7

1. Willett, W.C. and Ludwig, D.S., 2020, 'Milk and health', *New England Journal of Medicine*, 382(7), pp. 644–54.
2. Willett, W.C. and Ludwig, D.S. 2020.
3. Mac Mary, S., et.al. 2006, 'Assessment of effects of an additional dietary natural mineral water uptake on skin hydration in healthy subjects by dynamic barrier function measurements and clinic scoring', *Skin Research and Technology*, 12 (3), pp. 199–205.
4. Palma, L., Marques, L.T., Bujan, J. and Rodrigues, L.M. 2015, 'Dietary water affects human skin hydration and biomechanics', *Clinical, Cosmetic and Investigational Dermatology*, 8, p. 413.

Chapter 10

1. Khazdair, M.R. et al. 2015, 'The effects of *Crocus sativus* (saffron) and its constituents on nervous system: A review', *Avicenna Journal of Phytomedicine*, 5 (5), p. 376.

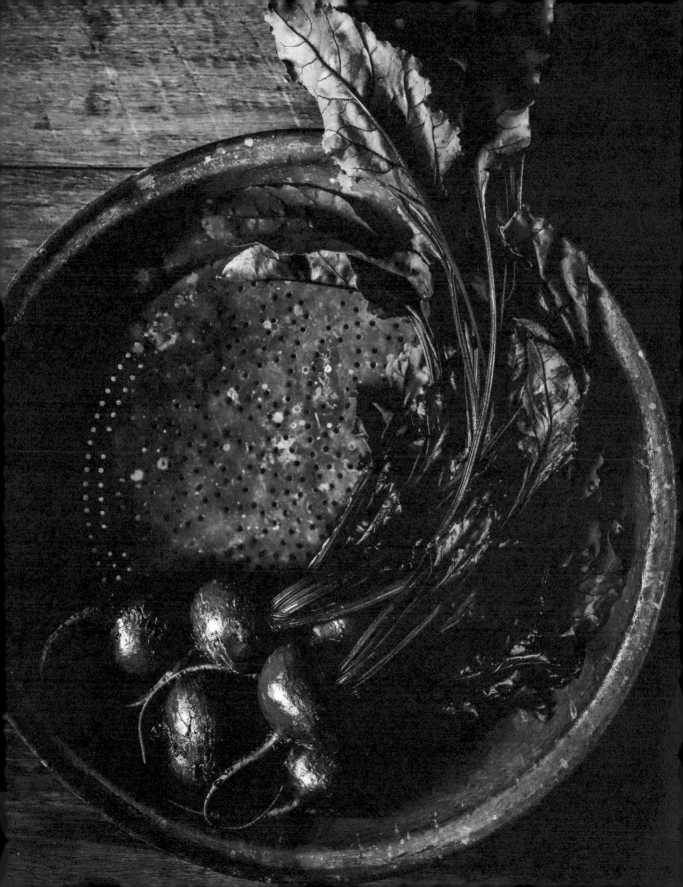

Recipe index

Index

COVID-19 pandemic 25
cow's milk 92
cravings, gut microbes 10–11
creams *vs* balms 69

D
dandruff 82
dermatitis 83
diamine oxidase (DAO)
    depletion 30–1
    increasing 33
diet, low chemical 2–3, 100
dry skin
    cooking oil options 92
    hydration 95
    signs, symptoms and solutions
      83

E
eating out 91
eczema
    cooking oil options 92
    signs, symptoms and solutions
      84
evening primrose oil 70

F
fasting
    author's first experience 14–15
    how to begin 15–16
    time limit 15–16
    tips 16
fasts
    best meals to break 17
    types of 13–14
fermented foods 3
firm and tone menu 98
fish
    to avoid 94
    healthy list 94
flaxseed oil 64
flaxseeds 37
food chemical chart 3
food chemical intolerance 2–3
Food Intolerance Diagnosis

Program (FIP) 107
frijoles negros 36
fruit, washing 13

G
glutathione 67
gluten debate 40, 42
gratitude
    good vagal tone 23
    relief of itching 84
gratitude therapy 24–5
green onions 45–6

H
hair loss 80
heart rate variability (HRV)
    testing 21
hemp milk 93
hemp seed oil 38
hidradenitis suppurativa 84
histamines
    diet low in 100–1
    sensitivity/intolerance 2–3
    sensitivity/tolerance 85
hives 85

I
ice-cream maker instructions 196
immune wellness 103
inflammation allergies, vagus
    nerve 21
instant oats 40
intermittent fasting 14
Irish oats
itching, relief of 84

J
juice, while fasting 13

K
keratosis pilaris 85, 98

L
laughter, benefits of 24

leaky gut 86
leeks 38–9
light sensitivity 86
linseeds 37

M
magnesium 58–9, 60, 61
mast cell activation syndrome
    (MCAS) 87
mental health, skin wellness 9
mercury-rich fish 94
microbiome
    damaging foods 12
    health tips for 13
    healthy foods for 11–12
    what is it 10–11
milks
    farmed 92
    oat 93
    options for skin types 92–3
    plant-based 92–3
    rice 93
mind–skin connection 19
molybdenum 66
mung bean sprouts 33–5
music, recommended 199

N
niacin 63–4
nicotinamide 63–4
nourish/detox menu 99

O
oat milk 93
oatmeal bath sock 70
oats
    colloidal oat powder 70
    general information 39
    steel cut 40
    types available 40, 70
obesity, sweet potato 46–7
oily skin, clear skin menu 97
omega-3 64–5
oven temperatures 107

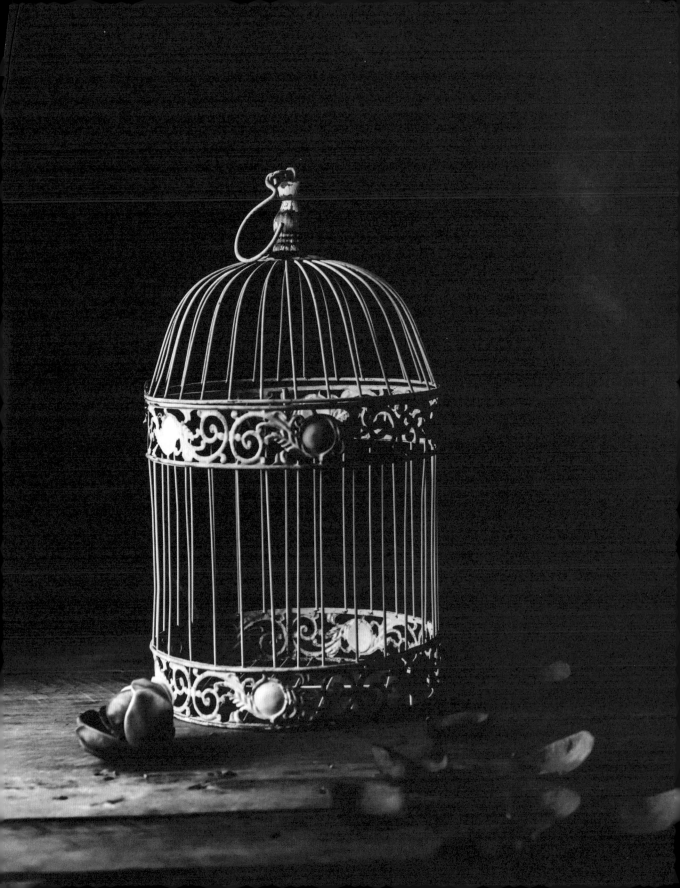